COMPREHENSIVE
BREAST CARE

And

Surviving
Breast Cancer

by

Dr. JOEL BERMAN

M.D., F.A.C.S.

BRANDEN BOOKS
Boston

Library of Congress Cataloging-in-Publication Data

Berman, Joel, Dr.
  Comprehensive breast care : surviving breast cancer /
  by Joel Berman.
    p.cm.
  Includes bibliographical references and index.
  ISBN 0-8283-2057-8 (alk.paper)
    1. Breast--Cancer--Popular works.
    2. Breast--Care and hygiene--Popular works.
    I. Title.

RC280.B8 B466 2000
616.99'499'03--dc21
            00-042943

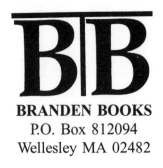

BRANDEN BOOKS
P.O. Box 812094
Wellesley MA 02482

Another book about the breast, the market's saturated!
But this one's different, quite concise, and not at all x-rated.
So pick it up and browse the chapters and you'll soon agree,
This is the west's best test bless'd breast book you will ever see.

Dr. Berman's Breast Book breaks all rules in its milieu
It's as easy to devour as a pot of Irish stew.
If you are in the mood to learn and have a pleasant read,
Turn just one page and that's enough for him to plant the seed.

A book on breasts doesn't have to be a dull and boring tome,
A blah recital of the facts to bury in your home.
The subject can be fascinating and a joy to share with friends,
For weddings and divorces or for other odds and ends.

The writer is a genius, and he's humble and refined
A breakthrough in the world of breasts, a mammary mastermind.
I understand he's just a surgeon (he cuts and doesn't think.)
It's safer for him to write a book (and cut carrots in the sink).

So buy his book and doing so, you'll save uncounted persons
(Because as years go by, a surgeon's knife skill only worsens.)
When else was it both a blessing and a grand profanity?
By purchasing this book you will be saving...humanity.

Finally a book about the breast, of mammary proportions
The author tells exciting tales without the least distortions
For twice the price you couldn't get its equal, none exists.
This is The Book on breasts, so cross all others off your lists.

To My Wife Andrea

and

To The Memory of My Sister Beth

*Who Died of Breast Cancer at a
Young Age*

So Many Years Ago

ACKNOWLEDGEMENTS

I am indebted to the many contributors who shared their expertise in writing parts or all of the following Chapters. The one thing which distinguishes this book from so many others is the input of many and widely differing points of view in different areas of breast care management. Chapter 9 on Lymphedema has a significant input from a Physical Therapist, Shari Fusco, who has specialized in the treatment of lymphedema, and is registered with the National Lymphedema Network. Chapter 13, a major treatise of Pathology, was primarily prepared by Pathologist, Dr. Kamini Malhotra, with input from her husband, Dr. Sheldon Barasch, also a Pathologist. In Chapter 14 on the Primary Care Physician's role, I was greatly helped by the input from Gynecologist, Dr. Terence M. O'Heany. Chapter 15 was the labor of Dr. David Cassidy and Dr. Stephen Simon, outstanding diagnostic and interventional Radiologists with a specialty in Mammography and Stereotactic Core Biopsy. In Chapter 16, I drew heavily on the experience of Dr. Lalita Pandit, who has taken specialized training in Genetics relating to Cancer, and is the Director of our Genetics and Risk Assessment Program. Lori Ash, Manager of Psychosocial Services For OCRCC, and the "Heart" of the Cancer Program, describes her key role in Comprehensive Cancer Care in Chapter 18. Chapter 19 is written by Nutritional Specialist, Jean N. French, presenting a host of fascinating topics in her area of expertise. Dr. Glen Justice, an Oncologist, Medical Director of the OCRCC, has been one of the inspirations in the development of the Cancer Center, and a personal inspiration to me by his caring, knowledge, and continuing intellectual curiosity. His input in Chapter 20 on Chemotherapy of Breast Cancer is a seminal contribution to this book. Dr. Bichlien Nguyen, an Oncologist, Associate Director of the Center for Breast Care at OCRCC, has been a strong partner in the Comprehensive Care Program, and has written significantly on Hormones and Breast Disease in Chapter 21. Dr. Haresh S. Jhangiani, Oncologist, and Director of the OCRCC Stem Cell Transplantation Program, has contributed Chapter 23 on Recurrent Breast Cancer. Dr. Robert J. Woodhouse, Director of Radiation Therapy at OCRCC, presents a fascinating article in Chapter 25 on Radiation Therapy. Dr. Malcolm D. Paul, Plastic and Reconstructive Surgeon, helped immeasurably in the writing of Chapter 28 on Plastic and Reconstructive Surgery of the Breast. Chapter 27 outlines the many services provided by the American Cancer Society for the patient with benign breast disease and breast cancer, and Joanne O'Heany has been the key individual in bringing this program into the OCRCC, making it a truly Comprehensive Program, presenting her views in this chapter. Lynn McBride, bubbling with warmth and caring, has presented her views as a Mammography Technician in Chapter 29, and Carole Metcalf, RN, who has assisted me in many surgeries as a specially trained RN First Assist, wrote the major portions of Chapter 31, The Operating Room Nurse Speaks Out. Dr. Sara Mylavarapu, an Anesthesiologist, prepared the delightful section on Anesthesia, Chapter 30. I want to thank Len Holreiser for his wonderful caricature of the Tumor Board. My appreciation to Carol Walling, who contributed outstanding photographs of mammograms and instrumentations for the chapters on Radiology, Radiation Therapy, and Sentinel Node. I wish to thank Chrystal Werner for her contribution to the chapter on Lymphedema. I am indebted to secretaries Wanda Atkinson and Lena Bodnar for their help and support over the year in preparation of this work. Faith and Adrian Van De Ree contributed many of the diagrams and artwork along with helpful comments and review of the manuscript. I also would like to express my appreciation to Marissa Saplala for typing and proofing the manuscript, and Quan M. Nguyen for providing computer expertise.

Finally, to my wife, Andrea Berman, RN, OCN, for her insightful Chapter 22 on the Infusion Center and for her constant support during the long process of writing this book, I am eternally grateful.

Joel A. Berman, M.D., F.A.C.S.

CONTRIBUTORS

This is a book on comprehensive breast care and I have attempted to bring to you the expertise of several specialists in their own fields. Rather than a body of information on various subjects, this approach makes it a reference of experts in a field which depends on drawing the best from the best in a comprehensive manner. Breast care and cancer diagnosis and treatment is no longer a "one man" job, and it is the combined, interactive efforts of the men and woman below that make it what it is today.

Lori J. Ash, MSW, LCSW, BCD; Manager of Psychosocial Services, Orange County Regional Cancer Center (OCRCC)

Sheldon Barasch, M.D., Pathologist, Director of Pathology, Fountain Valley Regional Hospital and Medical Center (FVRHMC)

Andrea Berman, RN, OCN, Oncology nursing in The Infusion Center, OCRCC

David L. Cassidy, M.D., Radiologist, Director of Outpatient Imaging Center, FVRHMC

Jean N. French, RD, CNSD, Clinical Dietician, FVRHMC

Shari Fusco, PT, CLT, FVRHMC

Len Holreiser, Artist, formerly with *Chicago Tribune*

Haresh S. Jhangiani, M.D., Oncologist, Director of Stem Cell Program, OCRCC

Glen R. Justice, M.D., Oncologist, Medical Director of OCRCC, and Clinical Professor of Medicine, USC Norris Cancer Center

Lynn McBride, RT, Mammography Technician, Center For Breast Care, Imaging Center, OCRCC

Kamini Malhotra, M.D., Pathologist, FVRHMC

Carole Metcalf, RN, FVRHMC

Sara Mylavarapu, M.D., Anesthesiologist, FVRHMC

Bichlien Nguyen, M.D., Oncologist, Associate Director of The Center for Breast Care, OCRCC

Joanne O'Heany, Volunteer Director, American Cancer Society Information Office at OCRCC

Terence M. O'Heany, M.D., Gynecologist, FVRHMC

Lalita Pandit, M.D., Oncologist, Director of Genetic Counseling, OCRCC

Malcolm D. Paul, M.D., Plastic Surgeon, Clinical Assistant Professor of Plastic Surgery, University of California, Irvine

Stephen Simon, M.D., Radiologist, Imaging Center, FVRHMC

Appreciation for Adrian and Faith Van De Ree

Carol Walling, R.N., RT, (M) CT (CV), RDMS, Manager of Diagnostic Services, FVRHMC

Chrystal Werner

Robert J. Woodhouse, M.D., Radiation Oncologist, Director of Radiation Therapy, OCRCC

PREFACE

Walk through this Center of Care for the breast,
We'll pause and we'll answer your every request.
We share all our knowledge and experience here
And make it a journey of joy, not of fear.

So come, take my book, and I'll lead you right through
The x-rays and treatment, you'll learn what we do,
To carry the message to women all ages,
Who are able to wend their way through all these pages.

It will be an odyssey, I hope you'll enjoy
Not too serious or dull, the tools we'll employ.
Listen to facts, don't be misled by rumor,
And we'll finish our journey with pleasure and humor.

One out of every eight to ten women in the United States will develop breast cancer at some time during her life. Many of you may say, "What a terrible way to start a book on breast care!". I look at this from a different perspective. Thirty or forty years ago, most women who presented to their physicians with breast cancer had a large mass, and the disease was diagnosed at a later stage with relatively poorer prognosis. Today, breast disease has come out of the closet of embarrassment and negative stigma, and with this public recognition comes earlier diagnosis, less radical treatment, and better prognosis and cosmetic outcomes. Development throughout the United States of "Centers For Breast Care" will lay the groundwork for the early diagnosis and treatment of breast diseases.

Although many subjects will seem academic, this is rather a book which will present a view of medical care for the woman of today who wants appropriate information and demands personal interaction which has often been lost and devalued in today's world in breast care. This approach towards a host of diseases and changes in the female breast lets a woman face her adult years with confidence and knowledge, and seek out medical advice and treatment at a center which can offer a comprehensive program of breast care with ancillary services which we now know should accompany that service.

An odyssey is defined as an extended wandering or journey...and that is what we are about to take. It is a very personal journey which starts with every female from the development of her body during adolescence. The breast plays a role in this development for it is often the first real sign of feminine change over which she has no control, and it is only after years of growth that she becomes aware that this agent of beauty, nursing function, and femininity has a problematic side, one of discomfort or concern over serious illness. In our next chapter, we will walk with you through a Center of Comprehensive Breast Care, and hopefully it will be a walk of knowledge and wisdom and through this to awareness and understanding.

But let me get back to my initial statement. One out of every eight to ten women in the United States will develop breast cancer at some time during their lives. Rather than being a depressing fact, this actually presents us with a very encouraging challenge. MOST OF THESE WOMEN WILL SURVIVE THEIR BREAST CANCER! What's the difference between the women of the 1920's and 1930's and the women of the 21st century? The cancer types they develop are probably the same; but the ability is now present to make early diagnosis when the tumor is very small. In the past, women had extensive operations as a standard of practice. The woman of today is encouraged to take advantage of the many diagnostic and physical examinations available to discover a tumor when it is very small and in its early stages.

While the operation (radical mastectomy) which Dr. William Halsted popularized in the 1890's remained the state of the art to cure breast cancer for more than fifty years, it is no longer the standard of practice, and it is no longer an acceptable mode of therapy for most women. Tumors of the breast were initially diagnosed by an examining physician; we now have diagnostic procedures which can detect lesions (abnormalities or cancer) on mammograms before anything can be felt on examination, diagnosing cancers that have not yet reached the potential to spread beyond the local area of origination. Women are now taught breast self-examination, and women from different countries and different cultural backgrounds who in the past never felt comfortable touching themselves, today have been taught how to do a monthly self-examination.

Under the aegis of Dr. Bernard Fisher, a leader in cancer research in America today, studies often involving many thousands of women were performed by the National Surgical Adjuvant Breast and Colon Program (NSABCP). These programs confirmed that breast preserving procedures such as the combination of lumpectomy, axillary dissection, and radiation therapy could be as effective in curing cancer as the very radical procedures originally outlined. Several chapters will go more into detail with these issues.

A few years ago, a patient came into my office with advanced breast cancer who had undergone several types of treatment but had recurrence of her disease. Many of the treatments had failed, and she had come to me to discuss some of the other options that she felt were available to her. She stated that she had received information from several clinics in Tijuana, Mexico, about different kinds of treatment of advanced cancer. My opinion of these programs was generally negative as many patients with cancer often seek alternative modes of treatment, and I also knew that a great number of these are ineffective, expensive, and unproven methods of treatment. I felt the "Tijuana clinics" were taking advantage of patients at what was often the lowest point in their lives, and I did not think that she should waste her money on these types of treatments.

A very bright young woman in her late thirties, the patient asked me what experience I had with alternative treatments, and whether I had any factual basis for my negative reaction to her proposals. I sheepishly admitted that I had not looked into the subject in detail, and I decided at that point to make a study of the alternative modes of practice in relationship to breast cancer treatment.

I had two of my office personnel write to several clinics in Tijuana asking for information about treatment for advanced breast cancer, and also wrote to the National Institute of Health and the American Cancer Society for information regarding the programs which are available and which were not in line with conventional treatments for breast cancer. To my surprise, I received a voluminous amount of literature from all sources. Those I received from the Tijuana Clinics were often sophisticated videotapes and literature emphasizing how these programs worked, with great attention being paid to the psychosocial aspect of the program--a warm loving demeanor of those people caring for patients, and emphasizing high cure rates, and quick reimbursement by insurance companies (a point which proved untrue in almost all cases). Suffice it to say, I ended up doing a comprehensive study of both alternative and complementary methods of cancer treatment, and I spend a chapter on this interesting subject, discussing the more prevalent drugs and treatments.

I have discovered that the one thing that was missing almost universally in the care of patients with breast cancer in the United States was a loving interaction between the patient and physician, a certain caring which we now know is encompassed by the all inclusive term of Psychosocial Approach to medical treatment. In 1825, Samuel Coleridge, the famous poet (remember "The Rime of the Ancient Mariner"?) stated, "Life without hope draws nectar in a sieve, and hope without an object cannot live." We will have more to say about the psychosocial approach to medicine in a future chapter; it underlines the heart of any "cancer program".

Therefore, let me introduce you to a Center for Breast Care. In the following chapters, we are going to explore various aspects of breast disease, diagnosis, and treatment, emphasizing that most diseases in the breast are NOT cancerous.

Let us begin our journey.

I wish my life were like a book, and not a jumble of nonsense,
And I could trace my future in a simple Table of Contents.
You see this book has the joy of knowing exactly what will come
next,
And it can follow its future just by looking it up in the text.

We often say a person's life is like an open book,
And yet you never have a chance to open it and have a look.
Because life is a mystery book, there's no Table of Contents to
find,
Each chapter opens another era, leaving the last behind.

I have to live life in a sequential order, I can't start out old, then
get young.
And "If I knew then what I know now" wouldn't be on the tip of
my tongue.
But you see, I can live the life of this book, and jump from "age"
to "age",
Merely by choosing the topic I want, and turning to that very
page.

CONTENTS

LIST OF FIGURES

Chapter 1
COMPREHENSIVE CENTER

Why in the world choose a name like that, the
"Comprehensive Center"
When a simple name like "Place For Women", or
"Breasts R Us" is better.
The intellectual set might well prefer a simple
"Amamus Mammae"
(The Southern sector would insist upon "Mammae Alabammae").

The Californians would label theirs--"Best Breasts in the West",
Chicagoans would go for "Breasts in the Loop" as best.
New Yorkers, of course, would always stick with "The Two
Big Apples"
And clerics would favor the spiritual side of "Mothering Mary
in the Chapels".

But whatever name we choose, consider the center
as comprehensive
No matter how the words come out, the treatment should be
extensive.
The problem is too many places just hide behind a name,
You should demand quite simply that what they do is
what they claim!

What is a Comprehensive Center for Breast Care?

I n today's fast-moving world, it is important to take a moment to reflect on the priorities in our lives. And most of them center around the assumption that we have goals and loves, and that we have family objectives. But perhaps the underlying basis for much of what we do is the assumption that our health will allow us to lead full and gratifying lives. It's not unnatural for a twenty to thirty-year-old person to assume a carriage of indefatigability and health. As many of us move into the forties with minor aches and pains of joints and backs and strained muscles, we also become more aware of our own place as physical beings. Those with the chronic diseases which have started in youth such as diabetes mellitus or asthma probably begin to look at health as a reality at an earlier age. But for most of us, at some time in our forties, a light of understanding suddenly is turned on which plays havoc with our previous belief of seeming immortality.

And such is the mindset and undefined thought of the forty-year-old woman who goes for her first mammogram, whether as a screening modality or because she has found a "lump" in her breast or at the recommendation of a physician.

My objective in this book is to present an approach towards breast health which is both informational and supportive to women and their families. It is not a comprehensive tome on the breast for a surgeon, oncologist, internist or family physician although many subjects will seem academic. It is rather a book which will present a view of medical care for the woman of today and her family, who want appropriate information, and demand a caring and personal interaction which have often been lost or undervalued in the medical world of today.

A Center for Breast Care will outline for you an approach toward a myriad of diseases and changes in the female breast so that a woman can face her adult years with confidence based on knowledge, and seek out medical advice and care at a Center which offers a comprehensive program of breast care with all the ancillary services which we now know should accompany this undertaking.

When a woman calls the Center for Breast Care (CBC), she arranges for an appointment for either a simple screening mammogram at the imaging center or opts for the complete comprehensive program. The comprehensive program is explained to her, and if she chooses this, an appointment is made, and she comes to the center at the arranged time. A clinical specialist is assigned to the woman who takes a limited, specific breast history which will include age of menarche (first menstruation), number of children and age at first pregnancy, number of previous biopsies, presence of lumps or previous cancer, and family history of breast disease. This information is rapidly placed in a small computer which can calculate her risks for developing breast cancer in her lifetime (see Gail Model Assessment).

The patient then goes for a mammogram under the expertise of specially trained mammography technicians who have instruction in psychosocial concerns as well as the techniques of breast mammography. The films are immediately read by a radiologist at the facility, and a decision is made whether further views or possibly an ultrasound study of the breast is needed (refer to section on radiology). This report is then given to the CBC physician who meets with the patient to discuss the findings briefly, and do a complete breast examination. The woman is instructed in the proper way to do self-examination of the breast, and questions are answered as they arise, in this regard.

Then fully re-clothed, she is sent to a viewing room where she can watch a videotape of breast self examination in her own language (usually at our center this means English, Spanish, Vietnamese and Chinese) along with a volunteer from the local chapter of the American Cancer Society (ACS) who can offer her a host of printed information on breast or other related topics.

The patient is then brought to the physician's office where she is accompanied by a member of our psychosocial service department as well as the ACS representative. The physician places her mammograms on a viewing screen, and explains to her the meaning of the various shadows, indicating the fatty tissue, supporting tissue, blood vessels, cysts and lumps, architectural abnormalities, microcalcifications and any other significant findings. If the patient wants to see what a cancer looks like on a mammogram, the physician may show her a film demonstrating this. The physician will give a brief natural history of the changes that occur in the female breast as she progresses in age, and give her an understanding why it is necessary for her to do monthly self-exams and yearly breast mammograms. (We recommend starting screening mammograms at age forty unless there is a strong family history of breast cancer or the presence of suspicious masses.) She is given information about the use of hormones and the importance of diet and an introduction to the genetic basis for breast cancer in some families. A silicone breast model with "lumps" in it is available for a patient to examine as a simulated breast lump while guiding her hands during the exam. She is asked to present any questions she may have about any aspect of the comprehensive program, and is referred to expert advice or other specialists for the complete answer. If abnormalities are found during her mammograms, the findings are rapidly discussed with her personal physician, and if the doctor agrees, we will discuss the finding and our recommendations with her. At some point in this process, the physician and ACS volunteer leave the room, and the woman has an opportunity to discuss any other issues with the social worker, who is specially trained in interacting with this type of situation, whether it be cancer or just psychosocial issues related to breast health.

It is stressed to each patient that breast care may be a one physician program until a cancer is diagnosed, at which time it becomes a team approach, offering her diverse specialists in the cancer field. It is much like having a second, third, etc., opinion all at once.

Every patient diagnosed with cancer is presented to a weekly "Tumor Board" of specialists consisting of oncologists, pathologists, breast surgeons, radiologists, radiation therapists, internists, family practitioners, nurses and social workers. Each case is presented with history, x-rays, and pathology slides, and a discussion ensues with the development of an appropriate course of action. The patient is not present at these discussions to allow a full uncensored flow of ideas and discussion which might be tempered by the presence of the individual. The recommendations are then presented to the referring physician and then to the patient.

Sometimes patients present to the center for second opinions and a similar program is followed. A strong emphasis is placed on the personal interaction between physician, patient, and psychosocial support individual, and the program has numerous support groups for helping a woman through her care and treatment should she be diagnosed with cancer.

The center focuses on the patient as an individual and stresses personal interaction, warmth and caring as well as a focus on accurate and understandable information. It is hoped that when she leaves the center, she will feel that her breast health has been handled in a complete and sensitive manner, making it an overall positive experience rather than one of fear and foreboding.

In the course of this book, we will progress through normal anatomy and physiology to breast examination, surgery, and a whole series of articles by specialists in each area. It is an attempt to condense a great deal of information into a usable reference for the woman of today.

Chapter 2
THE BREAST IN HISTORY
AND HISTORY
OF THE TREATMENT OF
BREAST CANCER

The female breast as an object of beauty and femininity has been reflected in painting and sculpture and described in literature for over 4,000 years. It has been revered as a symbol of fertility, sensuality, sexuality, and nurturing.

The *Venus* of Willendorf of 25,0000 to 20,0000 B.C. in the Naturhistorisches Museum in Vienna is a classic example of the nurturing breast from the earliest of historical figures. It is a 4-3/8" limestone carving showing a woman with large breasts and possibly pregnant.

Breasts have come to represent woman in the United States to a great degree. So it is not so strange that this "modified" sweat gland, the breast, is treated and regarded in a manner quite different from any other organ in the body. What it is and what it represents are so strongly integrated into our culture, that its mutilation or loss often threatens the very basis of the woman as an individual. With the American "ideal" of the full-breasted woman broadcasted in magazines, film, and television, no wonder there is a tremendous fear of loss and that it is perhaps way out of proportion to the loss of the organ itself. When a woman at age 40 enters the mammography center for the first time, she is consciously or unconsciously bombarded with the thoughts of potential tragedy and fear. As we continue through this book, the psychosocial approach to this very problem will be discussed instead of "sweeping it under the rug" as has been done for so many years.

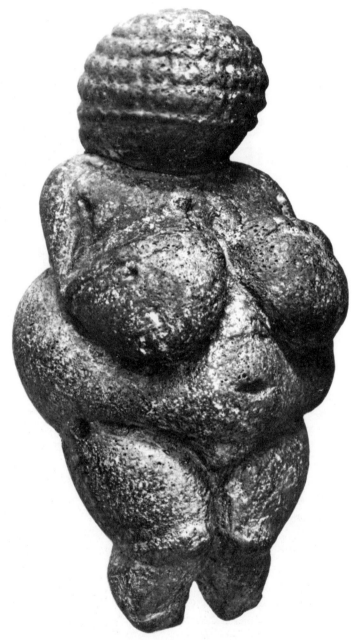

Figure 1. *Venus* of Willendorf (photo, courtesy of
Giraudon/Art Resource, NY).

The nude breast as a prominent figure in relationship is seen from ancient Egypt...

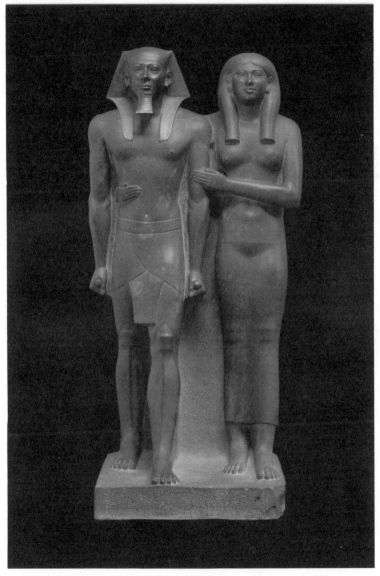

Figure 2. King Mycerinus and a Queen (photo, courtesy
of Museum of Fine Arts, Boston).

As well as in 20th century Yoruba maternity figure...

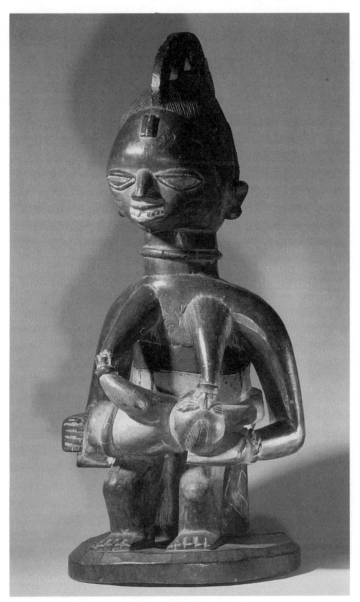

Figure 3. (photo, courtesy of Werner Forman Archive,
P. Goldman Collection, London)

During the 11th century, this was characterized as an "ideal woman"...

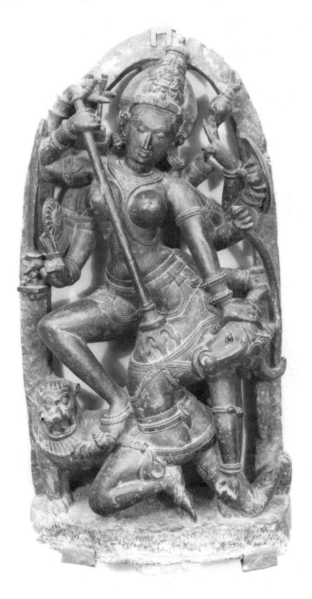

Figure 4. Durga, Medieval period, 11th century (photo,
courtesy of Giraudon/Art Resource, NY).

Note the nurturing figures of mother and child from ancient India depicting Yashoda and Krishna from 11-12th century...

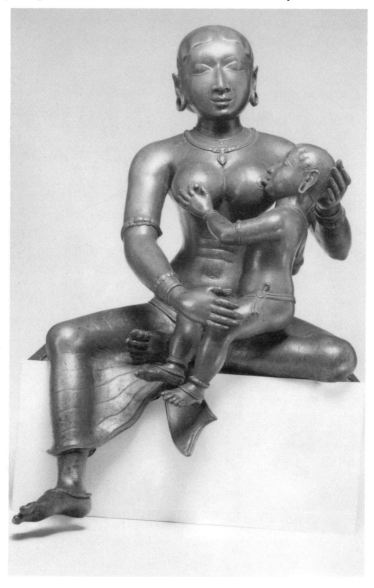

Figure 5. Yashoda and Krishna (photo, courtesy of
The Metropolitan Museum of Art, NY).

The "classical" woman's breasts are depicted throughout history from "Apollo and Daphne" by Gianlorenzo Bernini from 1622-24 to the famous "Kiss" by Auguste Rodin.

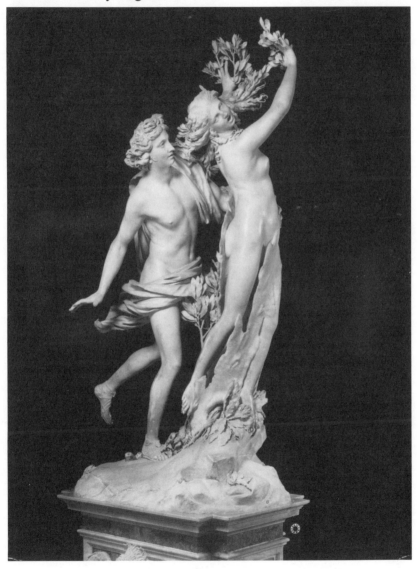

Figure 6. Apollo and Daphne (photo, courtesy of Alinari/Art Resource, NY).

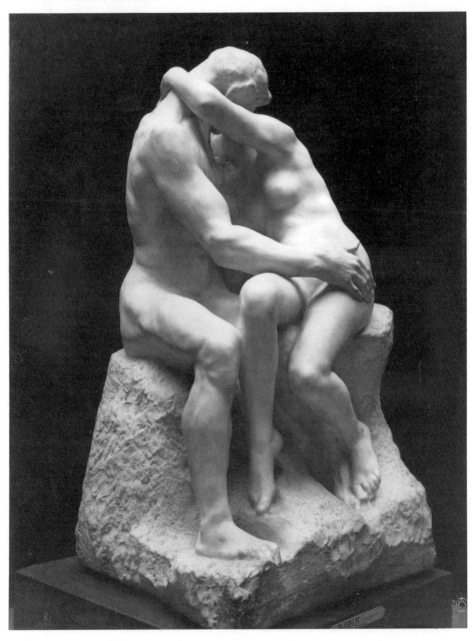

Figure 7. "Kiss" by Auguste Rodin (photo, courtesy of Archivi
Alinari/Art Resource, NY).

And even in the 20th century, the universal focus in the woman is often on the presence of her breasts whether in a classical or modernistic style...

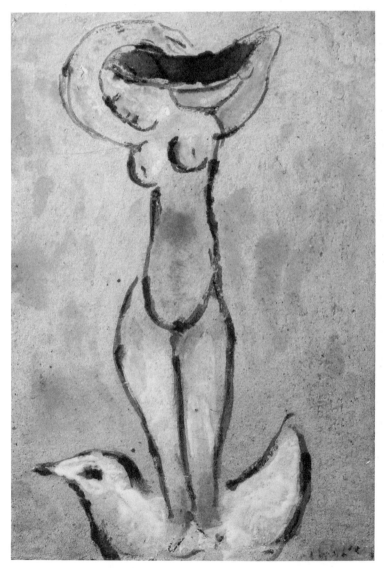

Figure 8. Woman by Marc Chagall (photo, courtesy of
Giraudon/Art Resource, NY).

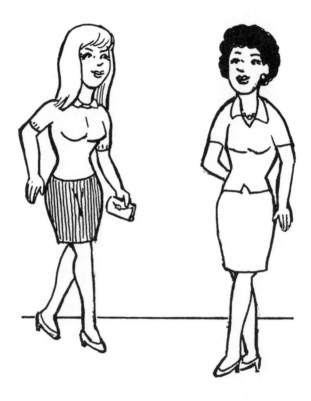

Figure 9. A 21st century woman by Len Holreiser.

In conclusion, I would like to present to you a poetic history of the management of breast disease which I gave recently, and which perhaps gives a more pleasant and palatable review of what might otherwise be a rather somber and depressing story:

HISTORY OF BREAST CANCER

I have come today to talk about a subject steeped in mystery,
The story of the human breast, as seen from ancient history.

The organ of which I want to speak is paired, unless bereft
Both men and women have just two, a right and also a left.
And diagnosis of a problem required no formality,
For simple sight and gentle touch revealed the abnormality.

In 1862, Edwin Smith traveled to Thebes (now Luxor) to be
specific,
And discovered a papyrus 15 feet long, which was written
in hieroglyphics.
Apparently scribed in 1600 BC, it described abscess, trauma,
and infection,
But in case #45 we find the earliest record of breast cancer
yet in detection.
The examiner is told about breasts with bulging tumors,
Cool to the touch and untreatable, and caused by
unknown humors.
The treatment proposed was burning with fire or removal with
instrumentation,
But there is no good record of any surviving one breasted
woman in that nation.

So let us proceed to old Babylon, 2000 years BC,
A Mesopotamian city of wealth, leisure and vice, headed by old
Hammurabi.
Initially physicians were scarce through the land,
For failure resulted in losing a hand.
The people were forced to find others in the marketplace with
similar afflictions for libations,

Thus the "whole of the people" was the physician,
the first "curbstone consultations".

Now the classical Greeks; We've all heard of old Socrates,
But how many know of the medic Hippocrates.
400 BC he described the four humors that lasted for quite a while,
One's blood, two phlegm, and the others the despicable yellow
and then the black bile.
He named the four elements - earth, air, water, and fire,
And that was the truth...don't call him a liar.
For health was the balance of all of the humors,
Without it, some sickened, some developed breast tumors.
Now Hippocrates told of three types of disease,
Which I list for you now, like a child's ABC's:
The first was disease he could cure with a medicine, the quashing
of illness, preservation of life.
The second not cured by the medicine, these required the use of
the knife.
And the third, and the worst, those not cured by the knife,
Required the fire to salvage their life.
And finally he stated, and in no uncertain terms,
That NO TREATMENT WAS BEST...THOSE TREATED OFTEN
ENDED UP IN MORTUARY URNS!!

From 150 BC to 500 AD The-Greco-Roman Period was
ushered to be.
A time when each home had its own household gods,
For the wealthy patricians or the beggars with hods.

Archagathus was known for his cruelty as surgeon,
And Leonidas cut breasts off with tumors to purge 'em.
Celsus, in 150 AD, described a breast cancer and went on to say,
A lot about surgical instrumentation which we've found
in Herculaneum and Pompeii.

And then we find Galen, 200 AD,
A giant of medicine for centuries to be.
Who wrote many volumes which were quite anatomical,

Some which we find today very comical.
His anatomy described ape, dog, pig, and cow rumen,
But he never studied the parts of the human.

He first described breast cancer, usually like a crab,
And taught purging and bleeding and excising the scab.
He described cures when tumors were completely excised,
If the cancer was local and not deep inside.

The medieval period was a time of great evil and chants,
Extending from Rome's downfall to the great Renaissance.
There was martyr and breast patron, Saint Agatha, so one hears.
Whose breasts were torn off with some dull iron shears,
For refusing the advances of the local governor,
who only wanted kisses for so deeply lovin' her.
We celebrate dear old Saint Agatha today
By carrying her breasts (two loaves of bread) on a tray.

In 1131 the council of Rheims made the rules,
Which led to the forming of the medical schools.
For they said no monks or clergy could practice the medicine,
And what a predicament that was to set us in.

But from 900 AD many Jews became physicians,
And wrote great tomes in many editions.
Moses Maimonides, a doctor to Saladin,
Wrote the Book of Council, and wrote of malade-in.

Rhazes, the father of Arabic medicine, was noted for excisions
of the breast,
And Ibn ben Abbas spoke of melancholic humors, and put
attitude to the test.
Avicenna, the "Prince of Physicians in Bahgdad" in 1005,
Wrote the Canon prescribing milk, diet, excision and cau-
tery...which left more dead than alive.
Albucasis in 1100 said, that small tumors when fully excised
had a place,
But he also admitted he never had seen a woman survive

such a case.
In conclusion this period was steeped in ignorance, horror, poor
results, and the absence of sages,
Perhaps that is why we will always recall it and call it
"Medieval Dark Ages".

Gun powder blew in the 15th century along with the
Gutenberg Press,
Then along came Vesalius with human anatomy, showing the
grand female breast.
The Renaissance blossomed with medical schools in Oxford,
Bologna, and Paris,
Ambrose Pare began tying off arteries, bleeding would many fewer
surgeons embarrass.
He excised simple tumors using pressure for bleeders.
And noticed the lymph nodes and described them to readers.

Born in 1509, Michael Servetus described lung circulation
and look what it brought,
He was burned at the stake for "the crime of honest thought".
But in the annals of breast cancer he did a muscle-ectomy,
The forerunner of the radical mastectomy.
William Fabre, a high German surgeon, used instruments
to compress the base of the breast,
So his knife amputated more painlessly and swiftly leaving
an open wound chest.
He also was first to remove the armpit nodes although how he did
it's a mystery,
But then so is much of the work surgeons did while their patients
screamed on through this history.
John Scultes invented many surgical instruments ligatures, needles,
and traction,
And Guillaume Houppeville did a mastectomy giving him great
satisfaction.

The Age of Enlightenment 1700's, was just a misnomer 'tis said,
For the doctors were steeped in erroneous teachings and most
of their patients were dead.

Cancer was the stagnation and coagulation of bodily fluids,
As close to the truth as the tomes of the druids.
Camper and Mascagni spoke of why you died of diseases with
general Decomposition, wastings and purgings.
And the century ended with division of services from the
old barber/surgeons to surgeons.
The Hunter brothers, William and John, LeDran Petit, and Heister.
Removed breasts like a guillotine,
Swift as a Phillistine.
Fast as the speed they could muster.
All in all pain and suffering were terrible,
Poor results, mutilations, all very unbearable.
The century closed with no great progression,
The number of surgeons went into recession.

Now let us go to the nineteenth century.
Medicine was freed from its stale penitentiary,
By the introduction of two monumental contributions,
Overshadowing four thousand years of ablutions.
The first by Morton, in 1846 was ushered in with nary a peep,
With his anesthesia the surgeon could operate while his patient
as finally asleep.
And then Joseph Lister, a proud British baron, described
in so many terms,
Antisepsis, the role of bacteria, or to us just germs, germs, germs.
This now allowed safer and better procedures for the interested
surgeon to test,
And James Paget and Charles Moore in the late 1800's were
removing the female breast.
It was still felt that sorrow and anger added to cancer morbidity,
And encouraging a cheerful attitude led to increase in
patient's felicity.

By the turn of the twentieth century, Philadelphia became
the center of medical learning;
With Pancoast and Gross and William Halsted, the fever
of progress was burning.
Halsted performed and described his mastectomies from beginning

to dénouement,
And breast cancer survival for the first time in four thousand
years, showed significant improvement.
For seventy years the radical mastectomy was held as the finest
for cancer of the breast,
To be followed by modified procedures whose results also met
the test.

And now we are focused on breast preserving procedures,
Which along with radiation, have similar long term cures.
And to these we've added the hormones and chemo-and
immunotherapy modes,
Depending a lot on the presence or absence of locally
involved nodes.

And now cancer can even be detected by x-ray so early,
that no mass is felt,
Which allows us to cure even more and more people, whose lives
this bad hand have been dealt.

And to continue I'd like to run through,
A somewhat complete, comprehensive review
Of the factors that have been put forth as the cause of cancer,
When people did not have a sensible answer.

The putrefying property of air, with stagnation and coagulation,
Pressure from garments, contusions, and bodily internal
derangement of fluids and libation.
And Astruc stated, and I quote the obsession:
"The complacency nowadays with which one allows ones teats to
be taken and handled, exposing them to compression."
Then frolicking with a husband, a trauma or hemorrhoid
or psychic depression were blamed,
A sedentary life which slackened the flow of bodily humors
was named.

And in conclusion we must run down a list of the agents
which centuries offered for cure,

Improved circulation, poultices, plasters, juice of nightshade,
                                          and tobacco
                    -- it seems like a sewer.
Lead and mercury ointment, frog spawn, rotten apples, veal
                              and pigeon, cut up in a paste,
Sulfur and vinegar, compress of urine, frog's meat,
                                    crawfish in a baste,
Secret remedies of nuns, garlic, milk, and toad broth,
The list is as endless as the troubles they wrought.

So be happy and cheerful when you walk in my office,
And see no vials filled with slugs or urine or crawfish.
For I'll just recommend modern methods and cures,
Thank you, good day, I'm sincerely yers,
               Doctor Joel Berman

Chapter 3
ANATOMY
OF THE FEMALE BREAST

Anatomy was at its best
When Neanderthal discovered the breast
And Vesalius was first to note
That little thing hanging in your throat.

But we've more important things to see
To pass down to posterity
We must show medical students the roads,
Of ducts, lobules, nipples, and nodes.

I'll give you a brief but adequate story,
(Not too gross and not too gory)
So you will know the veins and arteries
And be able to speak at cocktail parteries!

S ince I am not writing this for medical students, it is inherent upon me to give a simple yet complete enough presentation so that the major areas of interest and importance are covered. I was initially going to have a separate page entitled "The Normal Female Breast", but then I realized that there is no such thing. We all recognize that there is a multiplicity of sizes and shapes to the "normal" female breast, and it is each age and each society that determines what is its own ideal. The ideal to the average European, Asian, African, or Eskimo is quite different from that of the "American", and the preferences of the 21st century are quite different from the 1920's, so we won't necessarily use the term "normal" breast with regard to appearance but there are basic structures to the breast with which we must be familiar.

The mammary gland or breast, strictly speaking, is a modified sweat gland (sorry, ladies), and is used for the nourishment of an infant. That it has psychosocial and physical appearance importance is another issue entirely. It is important to know embryologically that there is a "mammary line" that extends roughly from the axilla (armpit) to the groin (inguinal area) along which accessory (extra) nipples and accessory breast tissue may occur in development. Of course, breasts usually occur where they're supposed to, but some women have accessory or extra nipples. Some may have extra breast tissue, such as an increased bulging in the armpit which may get larger and smaller during the menstrual cycle, and occasionally cause discomfort, requiring removal of the extra breast tissue.

The female breast doesn't change much from infancy to puberty, but then there is an enlargement due to an increase in glandular tissue and fat. After onset of menses (menstruation), the breast will change during the month, enlarging during the premenstrual phase of the gland, and regressing in the postmenstrual phase.

During pregnancy, the breast enlarges after the second month, and there is increasing pigmentation and enlargement of the nipple complex. After the pregnancy and after the nursing period, the gland regresses and actually has a slight decrease in size, and becomes more flabby and pendulous. In the postmenopausal woman, the breast may regress to a smaller size consisting primarily of fatty tissue unless the woman is taking hormone medication.

Just to be complete, let me say that underdeveloped, overdeveloped, and inequality in the size of the breasts can occur, and usually doesn't become a problem unless the occurrence is extreme. Plastic surgical procedures are available after appropriate counseling and discussion with a physician and, if relevant, with the family. You may be interested to know that occasionally men can have unilateral or bilateral breast enlargement called gynecomastia, and this too may need surgery for emotional reasons, especially in teenage boys who may get teased in the locker room.

But let us progress to the basic anatomy of the breast so that when we talk about normal and abnormal findings in the breast, it will have more meaning. The gland (breast) may be slightly larger on one side, as mentioned before, and usually it is the left breast. It is composed of about 15 to 20 segments or lobes arranged in a circular or radial fashion around the nipple, and each lobe has its own tube or duct ending and exiting at the nipple. The breast also has some supporting tissue in the surrounding tissue called suspensory ligaments or Cooper's ligaments (what a thing to be immortalized for!) which add some elevating support to the gland. The breast may contain 50% or more fatty tissue, depending on individual differences. The area surrounding the nipple is called the areola, and under this there are glands (of Montgomery) which secrete a fatty material which lubricates and protects the nipple during nursing.

Muscle tissue in the areolar complex can cause the nipple to become erect in response to nursing or other stimulation. It is also important to know that many women have normally inverted nipples which is of no concern unless a normal everted nipple changes into an inverted nipple, as we shall learn in a later chapter.

Underlying the breast against the chest wall are two large muscles, the Pectoralis Major and the Pectoralis Minor. These muscles were routinely removed in the past when women underwent the old radical mastectomy procedure, but we rarely need to do this today (only when a cancer has extended to involve these muscles, they need to be removed to get rid of the entire cancer).

Lymph nodes, shaped like tiny kidney beans, are found throughout the body. They are also found in relationship to the breast. Their function is to drain lymph and waste from the breast tissue, and may act as an immunological barrier to some tumor spread. Their function has been explained by a pathologist. The diagram shows the areas in which lymph nodes are found in relationship to the breast, and we can see that the primary area of concern for the breast surgeon is the axilla or armpit. If breast cancer cells have spread to the lymph nodes in the axilla, there is a greater chance that they have spread elsewhere in the body. That is why we sometimes need to know whether lymph nodes are positive (involved with cancer cells) or negative in order to plan appropriate treatments. Some surgeons will talk of Level One, Two, and Three lymph node dissections, and this merely refers to the position of the nodes in relationship to the axillary vein (*see* diagram). In addition, we will talk in a later chapter about the sentinel, or first lymph nodes draining in any particular area of the breast.

There are several nerves we should consider when talking about the breast. Of course, there are the many tiny sensory nerves (nerves for feeling) which supply the breast tissue and the skin, and these are frequently disturbed during any type of breast surgery. Sensory nerves will regenerate in time although sensation will usually be different than previously. A sensory nerve that runs across the axilla, called the intercostobrachial or first intercostal nerve, supplies feeling to the back of the axilla and upper arm as shown.

Two motor nerves (nerves that innervate muscles and are needed for motion of that muscle) are important for us to know about. The long thoracic nerve supplies the serratus muscle, and the thoracodorsal nerve supplies the latissimus muscle. We will talk more about these in the chapter on surgery (axillary dissection).

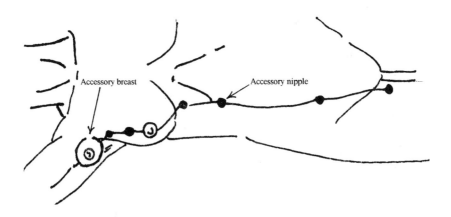

Figure 10. THE MILK LINE.

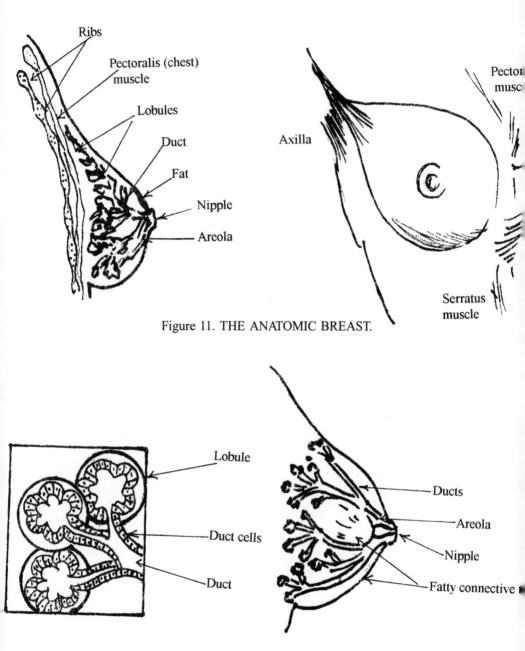

Figure 11. THE ANATOMIC BREAST.

Figure 12. MICROSCOPIC BREAST.

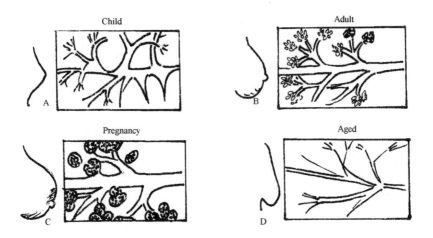

Child

Adult

Pregnancy

Aged

Figure 13. THE BREAST AT DIFFERENT STAGES.

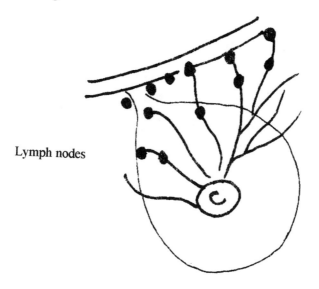

Lymph nodes

Figure 14. THE BREAST AND CHEST WALL.

Chapter 4
PHYSIOLOGY OF THE BREAST

You probably think I have some gumption
To tell you of your own body function
You don't really have to know the ilk,
Of having babies and producing milk.

But if you want to fight breast cancer
It's sometimes easier to find the answer,
If you understand the workings of the gland,
To take the situation full in hand.

We'll talk about what makes girls and boys
(And why they play with different toys)
It's not a secret of the Druids,
Its just those precious bodily fluids!

HOW IT WORKS

I'm just going to touch briefly on physiology of the breast because the effects of hormones will be covered in another chapter in relationship to cancer of the breast. But it is important to have a little information in these areas; the development of the breasts, the lactation process (production and secretion of milk), and the effects of natural estrogen and progesterone on the breasts.

The breasts of males and females are identical in young children, and are therefore what we call secondary sexual characteristics (unlike the genitalia which are definitely male or female at birth). Under the influence of certain hormones in the first decades of life, even a male breast can develop sufficiently to produce milk much like the female breast. It is natural estrogen in the female at the time of puberty that causes deposition of fat in the breasts and along with progesterone, causes the development of the various other areas of the breast such as the lobules and the ducts. Estrogens contribute to making the characteristic appearance of the adult breast. However, during pregnancy, the large amount of estrogen and progesterone secreted actually inhibits milk production until after the baby is born.

Progesterone, another naturally occurring hormone, promotes the final development of many of the breast structures. It is also responsible for the changes in breast size during the monthly cycle due to increased fluid collection in breast tissue, and can cause the recurrent pain and swelling of the breasts.

Although not generally mentioned to the lay public, a substance called growth hormone produced in the brain is also required for estrogens to produce their effect on the breasts.

And finally, just a few words on lactation (milk production). By the end of pregnancy, the breasts have been prepared by the body for production of milk but this does not come to fruition until after the baby is born. The initial fluid called colostrum contains lactose and proteins and almost no fat and is very minimal in volume. Remember, it is the huge output of progesterone and estrogen produced by the placenta (afterbirth) during pregnancy that inhibits the massive flow of milk. When the placenta is gone after delivery, there is a secretion of another substance, lactogenic hormone (prolactin), by a part of the brain (called the adenohypophysis) which causes the breast to secrete copious amounts of milk rather than colostrum.

And still another hormonal system comes into play to allow the milk to flow down the ducts and out the nipple into the baby's mouth. When a baby sucks, it causes a stimulation which in turn causes the release of other hormones called oxytocin, and to a smaller degree, vasopressin which induce milk ejection. Complex but interesting! And it is the continuous suckling that causes continued lactogenic hormone production and continued milk. Therefore, if a woman stops nursing, the hormone will stop and in a couple of weeks milk production will cease. Obviously, this is a very simplified description of what happens, but it gives you a basic understanding of the complex interaction of hormones effecting the female breast. And it should be emphasized that the development and function of the breasts is dependent upon many other hormones and body chemicals for normal processes to occur such as those produced by glands such as the thyroid, and another called the parathyroid which is responsible for calcium regulation in the body. The adequacy of a woman's milk production will also depend upon her maintaining a good diet to offset the losses from breast feeding, and this is why pregnant women and post-partum women are kept on balanced diets, and with vitamin and mineral supplements.

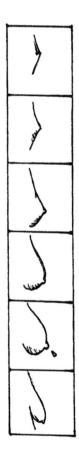

Figure 15. DEVELOPMENT OF THE BREAST.

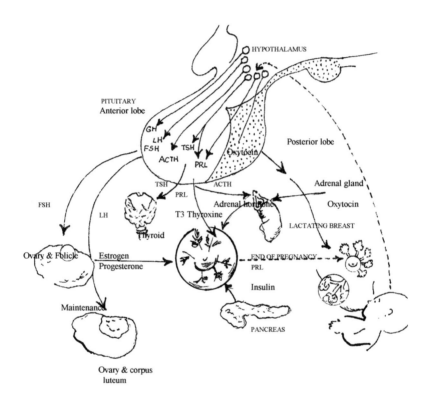

Figure 16. PHYSIOLOGY OF BREAST DEVELOPMENT
PHYSIOLOGY OF LACTATION

Chapter 5
BREAST EXAMINATION
AND SELF-EXAMINATION

I've got to do my breast exam,
My doctor said to do it.
I used to never give a damn,
I'd always just poo poo it.

But then my doctor found a lump,
He showed me how to feel it.
I had to have a mammogram,
And that would help reveal it.

My lump turned out to be benign,
I should have found it sooner.
And now I always check my breasts,
To palpate for a tumor.

One of the greatest advances in the early diagnosis of abnormalities of the breast has come in the area of breast examination. The physician has been trained for years in the careful manual examination of the breast and the axilla (armpit), and it has only been recently that a strong program of breast self-examination has been developed by doctors, by breast centers, and by vigorous programs such as that of the American Cancer Society and many other private organizations.

It is generally recommended that all women begin having yearly screening mammograms at age forty unless there is a strong family history of malignant breast disease. However, all women from their teenage years on should be aware of changes that can occur in their breasts, and should learn breast self-examination at a young age. We will go into a more detailed description of the exam itself, but it must be mentioned at the outset that MOST LUMPS FELT IN THE BREAST ARE NOT CANCER. Many women fear doing self-examination because they are afraid of what they may find, and as silly as this may sound, there are many women who just don't want to know what's going on until it becomes more problematic. It's the "If I ignore the exam, maybe nothing will happen" philosophy to which we all fall guilty at some time or other. But women have now become aware of the importance of self-examination, and with the encouragement of their physicians, family members, and breast centers, a whole new vista has opened in this area. Even women who have never felt comfortable touching their own breasts for cultural or psychosocial reasons have now "come out of the closet", and started taking personal responsibility for their own breast health. In many Asian cultures, it is not considered appropriate even for physicians to examine breasts, much less have the women examine themselves.

But enough for background. There are many ways to examine the breasts, and any of the accepted methods are okay if a woman practices and becomes somewhat expert in the method she chooses. She should examine her breasts once a month and preferably at the same time each month. Put it on the calendar as part of the monthly routine. And in some women, who have times during the month when the breasts are very tender, avoid those times, and try to do the exam when there is the least amount of discomfort. Each woman will learn to know her breasts and after awhile will be able to identify abnormalities as they may occur.

Now about the examination itself. Depending on the body habitus (size and shape), a woman may be more comfortable doing an exam lying in bed, standing, or in the shower or bath. But the basic exam is the same. Using the flat of the fingers, not the fingertips, and not squeezing the breast between thumb and fingers, gentle pressure is placed on the breast first superficially and then more deeply, progressing around the breast so that no area is missed. This should also include the nipple and areolar area. In thinner women, a series of firm lumps may initially be felt, and these may be the ribs as they course around the chest under each breast.

When the breast exam is completed, the hand is pressed gently into the axilla (armpit) to feel for any lumps or tenderness.

Remember, most lumps felt are not cancer. But what do we feel? In young women and women on hormone replacement, the breasts may be very firm, and no definite masses or lumps can be found. Women during pregnancy and post-partum during nursing will have engorged breasts, also very difficult to examine (even for a trained physician). As a woman gets older, the breasts become more fatty and much easier to examine. God's gift to women--as they get older and into the higher risk age groups, its easier to find small lumps in softer, older breasts.

What happens in the breast that causes change, and how do we know what's important or not? I'm frequently asked this question, and these are some of the answers I have given. The normal breast goes through changes with aging, and these changes may be different with each individual. Some women will develop many cysts, and these will be followed by her physician and by x-rays or ultrasounds (*see* chapter on X-rays); she will learn to recognize these changes in her breasts. It is not uncommon for women, especially younger women, to develop a rubbery non-cancerous growth called a fibroadenoma which is rounded and moveable, and only needs to be removed if it is bothersome or rapidly increasing in size. Also, some women may have only a few large cysts which also are usually round and may be tender. When confirmed on x-ray, these can usually be drained by a physician using a needle.

While not always a definite finding, a cancer in the breast is usually irregular, very hard, and sometimes causes dimpling of the overlying skin, retraction of the nipple, an orange-peel appearance of the skin or tenderness. Needless to say, any new lumps in the breast should be seen by a physician and again, most will not be cancerous.

So, to recoup, we do a monthly self examination looking for lumps, any changes in the breast appearance, pain, skin and nipple changes, any nipple discharge (except during nursing) and any significant swelling not usual for that individual. The most important thing is to recognize the need to examine and follow-up with a physician if any abnormalities are present.

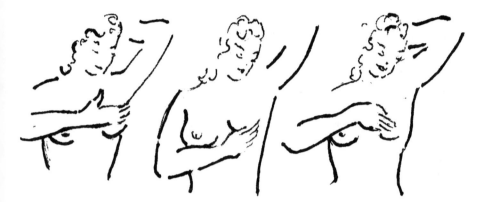

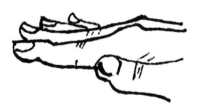

Use the flat of the fingers to examine, not the fingertips.
Go around the breast, applying gentle pressure.

Figure 17. BREAST SELF EXAMINATION.

Chapter 6
SURGERY OF THE BREAST

It takes a lot of arrogance
To wear a surgeon's pair of pants.
We're noted for our ego strength,
A humble lot, we certainly ain't.

But we love our work, with breasts and veins,
(As children we built model planes!)
And we derive great joy and pride,
In looking at you from inside.

Women surgeons, some say, are best,
For operating on the breast.
But I think the men are equally blessed
To pass a breast incision test.

In the surgical arena, ladies and gents,
What you really want's experience.
In the world of the surgeon
You don't want a virgin.

Surgery is one of the most frightening words a woman will face after she has been told she has an abnormality in her breast. Until then the whole workup, including examination and diagnostic procedures, has been minimally invasive, and somehow the reality does not "hit" the individual as strongly as the word surgery itself. It implies letting someone else actually take complete control, probably having to go to sleep, and having an incision made in the breast. It is often the last insult to the emotions, and frequently brings tears to a patient as I am explaining the procedure in question. Physicians and surgeons who have been involved in this for many years may sometimes lose awareness of the overwhelming nature of this undertaking to the average person, and thereby be insensitive to the psychological impact of surgery. Suffice it to say, it is a subject which I have to breach carefully, and with a constant reminder of what the individual is going through.

When a patient comes to me for breast surgery, I always sit down in my office and begin to explain the background and the procedure in as relaxing a fashion as possible. Your doctor should not treat you as an "inanimate" object, as a "breast" or a "disease entity", but as a feeling, emotional person, to allay all the natural fears which arise at this time; you can demand this type of approach or seek out another expert. If a doctor is too busy to spend the time, no matter how good or famous he may be, he's probably not the one for you!

But let's assume you have a considerate, charming, capable guy like me and you've just been told you need some type of surgery on your breast. Before we get into the specifics of the surgery you need, let's cover some of the things you will encounter prior to the surgery.

First of all, one of your physicians needs to do a complete physical examination to be sure that you are physically able to undergo the procedure, and if there are problems, correct them before progressing any further. For most surgery, a compete blood count (CBC), urine analysis, and a chest x-ray are required. In women over forty, I usually require an electrocardiogram (EKG) as a baseline evaluation of heart function, and I rely on the family physician to tell me about any special problems of which I should take special note. Patients with diabetes mellitus or high blood pressure (hypertension) need to have these conditions under control before surgery, and this can be accomplished fairly rapidly. Other blood tests may be indicated, and this will differ from patient to patient. Certain precautions are also advised in the preoperative (time before the surgery) period such as avoiding aspirin and other medicines which may cause increased tendency to bleed or "ooze", and patients on anticoagulation (such as Coumadin) for some other medical problem must have these temporarily stopped before the surgery.

We will go into detail with each procedure, but in general, a few things should be understood. Your surgeon should tell you in detail about the operation starting with the type of anesthesia (local--giving injections while you are partly or completely awake; general--when you are completely asleep - *see* the chapter on Anesthesia), describing how the medicine is given, and how you will feel before and after the procedure. Surgeons sometimes forget that the woman going for her first breast operation is often a novice to this whole milieu, and will appreciate any and all information offered to make it a less scary undertaking. The surgeon should draw pictures or show you a picture or diagram of your procedure, and indicate what kind of a scar to expect, and how long the healing process will be. And don't be afraid to ask about how much surgery of this type your surgeon does, and what the complications could be. We surgeons are sometimes "legends in our own minds", and too quick to acknowledge that complication is a word which all normal human beings must accept as part of being human.

Of course, the well trained, experienced physician will offer the best chance for an uneventful operation, but the confident surgeon never shies away from giving the patient a realistic view of the procedure in a reassuring, comfortable manner. The surgeon who says, "I've never had a problem or complication", in my estimation, is a surgeon to be wary of We will go into more detail about the potential complications of surgery in a later chapter, but every surgeon knows that he must weigh the risk of the operation with the health of the patient. "The operation was a success but the patient died" hardly needs be emphasized.

So let me begin by saying that in breast disease, we are trying to get away from procedures which need anesthesia and an operating room setting, as much as possible. Whereas years ago patients with a lump or abnormal mammogram needed surgical intervention, many of these procedures have become antiquated or completely unnecessary. Infections and some small abscesses can usually be treated in the physician's office, and most masses and radiological findings can be assessed and diagnosed prior to the need for a definitive operation. With the advent of the fine needle aspiration and then the core needle biopsies (which are done in a physician's office or radiological suite with a local anesthetic), very few patients need to have an open breast biopsy for diagnosis. You should not hesitate to discuss this with your doctor, and be ready to seek out a second opinion if it doesn't sound right to you. As I will discuss in the Comprehensive Breast Center, decisions are usually made by a "team", and when decisions come under the scrutiny of the "team", the treatment will usually be the best and the most conservative.

There is only one emergency which is truly surgical, and that is hemorrhage. (Don't get me wrong; of course, cardiac arrest and respiratory [breathing] failure are emergencies, but they are medical, not surgical.) All I want to emphasize is that if a surgical patient is bleeding, you have to "jump in", and do something right away. So remember this when you see a physician or surgeon about your breast problem. It's not an emergency! Even if you have a cancer, it has been growing probably for years, and a few days or weeks are not going to make any difference in the eventual outcome. Now the only exception I would make would be a breast abscess or infection where treatment should be started urgently, but again, it's not a life or death matter. Aside from this, no one should rush into a biopsy or operation until all the prerequisites mentioned above have been done, and until you are comfortable with the physician, the management, and the procedure recommended. If someone is in a hurry, just step back, and take a little inventory of the situation.

Now the reason we emphasize the needle or core biopsy is because this can frequently give us a diagnosis. Most very young women (teens and twenties) may have lumps, and if they are of questionable nature, may need a needle biopsy. These are usually benign, and no further surgery is indicated. Years ago, everyone was taken to surgery and had a resultant scar which today we know is unnecessary. If the needle or core biopsy is inconclusive (not enough cells are seen or the tissue seen cannot be satisfactorily evaluated by the pathologist), then an open biopsy may be indicated. Also, if a positive biopsy for cancer is found, the "team" can discuss the case and devise a treatment plan. We will discuss the "team" in another chapter, and show how this offers each patient a second, third, fourth, etc., opinion about her case which may be more comforting than relying on just one person for advice. (It's also good for the surgeon because it gives him backup support for the decision to operate and what procedure to do.) Cancer treatment is a team effort!

The patient should be told about where the incision will be, what type of scar to expect, and what type of sutures are used (the type that need to be removed, the type that don't [absorbable], or metallic skin staples). If the patient has a history of forming thick, unsightly scars (keloids), the surgeon should explain what to expect, and what he can do to minimize the scar (sometimes steroids can be injected to decrease the scar formation). After surgery, the patient will have incisional pain (where the operation took place), and will need to be informed about this, and reassured that her pain needs will be addressed appropriately. Many surgeons use a local anesthetic in conjunction with the general anesthetic so that the patient will have less pain when she awakens. For the immediate postoperative period, intravenous (in the vein) or intramuscular (in the muscle) injections are given to allay the more severe discomfort. Later, an oral medication (pill or capsule) may suffice.

In order to prevent an accumulation of blood in an operative site (inside the breast under the incision), many surgeons place drains in the wound for short periods of time (one to five days). These may be rubber strips (Penrose drains) or tubes connected to a small reservoir (such as Jackson-Pratt or Hemovac drains). Usually these are sewn in place, and safety-pinned to prevent them from either falling out or "falling in" to the wound. Some patients will be sent home with the drains which are then removed in the physician's office. Don't be surprised if there is some bloody drainage That means the drains are doing their job and "draining". Of course, as we will discuss later under "Complications", if bleeding is excessive, you need to contact your surgeon immediately.

Remember, when you have breast surgery, whether it is a small biopsy or a very extensive procedure, there will be varying degrees of deformity. There will always be some disfigurement, even if very minimal. You can't take something away from the breast and have it look exactly as before. Your surgeon should give you a good idea what to expect so there are no surprises after the procedure. And I must emphasize that breast preserving procedures are designed to leave the woman with a pleasing cosmetic outcome. If a surgeon does an extensive breast surgery, and "saves the breast" but ends up with a very marked cosmetic deformity, this may not be as good as doing a total mastectomy, and then having a plastic surgeon do a good reconstruction. The patient must ask the surgeon about these issues before the surgery.

Surgery not only causes cosmetic deformity, it also may change some of the sensations in the breast. Surgery of or near the areola and nipple may significantly alter the sensations felt when touched. With any breast surgery, it is not uncommon to have varying periods of mild to moderate discomfort which usually subsides in a few days or a few weeks. Sometimes a woman may experience occasional sharp or shooting pains in her incision either from scar tissue or from the regrowth of tiny sensory (feeling) nerves that must be cut during any surgery. Usually all these postoperative pains resolve with "tincture of time", and only rarely does a woman have persistent pain which requires a "nerve block" (injection of the area with medicine to deaden the nerves).

After most of my breast surgery, I wrap the woman's chest circumferentially with a very tight Ace bandage to prevent postoperative bleeding, and I usually leave this dressing in place for a day or two, advising her to loosen it if it is too constricting. I find this leads to fewer bleeding complications. Somehow, no matter how careful the surgeon, an occasional small blood vessel wants to start bleeding several hours after surgery, and the tight binding is a firm reminder to this little blood vessel, "Don't even think about it!".

Well, let's get down to the actual surgical procedures.

Abscesses

A cut is made into the abscess, and the infected material is washed out. This wound cannot be closed, and must be "packed" (have some string-like material placed) or have a drain placed. When the infection has resolved, it will either close on its own or a surgeon can close it secondarily (later closure as opposed to primary closure--closing it at the time the cut is made).

Simple excisions

Simple excisions are used for removal of benign (not cancerous) lumps such as fibroadenomas or recurrent cysts (cysts may be aspirated and may recur, even though not cancerous, and may need to be surgically removed). We also use simple excision for removing cancer which has recurred in a prior incisional area to sample the tissue (for appropriate later treatment), or to prevent skin breakdown, pain, bleeding or infection.

Open Biopsy

When a needle or core biopsy is insufficient or cannot be done, this procedure is performed. (Sometimes a woman has very small breasts, and the core biopsy apparatus cannot be used because there is not enough surrounding tissue, and the biopsy needle could actually injure or penetrate the chest wall. Sometimes the location of the mass to be biopsied is in an area of the breast which cannot be reached by the biopsy apparatus – i.e., too near the axilla or too far posterior near the chest wall. In patients with breast implants, a needle biopsy is not indicated for risk of penetrating the implant and requiring it to be replaced!) If possible, the surgeon prefers to make the incision around the areola so that the scar will be very minimal, but many times this is not possible, and an incision has to be made in the area of the breast where the abnormality is located. Surgeons are very aware of the need to keep the incision away from the upper portion of the breast which may show when a woman wears a blouse or bathing suit, or other more revealing garment. Make sure you ask!

There are two types of situations in which we can do a biopsy; one, where a mass can be felt, and the second, where there is no mass felt. In the first instance, the surgeon will make a small cut into the breast, and controlling any bleeding with electrocautery and by tying off bleeding vessels, remove the mass, and send it to the pathologist. The second is more difficult. This patient must first go to the x-ray department for what is called a "needle localization" of the area in question. As described in the "Radiology" chapter, one or more fine needles are placed in the area of abnormality (after a local anesthetic has been administered) using x-ray or ultrasound guidance (like having another mammogram or ultrasound). The patient is then sent to surgery with the needles in place, put to sleep, and has the tissue marked by the needles removed by the surgeon. This tissue is then sent back to the x-ray department (patient is still asleep) and the specimen is x-rayed to make sure that the surgeon has removed the lump in question. If not, further excision is needed; if successful, then the entire specimen is sent to the pathologist who may do a quick analysis (frozen section) or a permanent section (overnight analysis---better slides take more time to process--*see* "Pathology").

What is done after the biopsy is determined by what has been planned pre-operatively. If the mass is benign, usually no further surgery is needed. Sometimes the surgeon will only do a biopsy, regardless what is found, and discuss the findings with the patient. However, sometimes he will progress to the next operation to be described--the lumpectomy (segmentectomy, quadrantectomy, partial mastectomy--all the same surgery varying only in degree).

Lumpectomy

A lumpectomy is just what it says--removal of a lump. Usually this is done for cancer, and we always want to remove the entire cancer along with a margin of non-cancerous tissue ("the free margin"). How wide to make this margin is argued from surgeon to surgeon; I prefer at least one centimeter or more to feel comfortable that I have "gotten around" the tumor, but many very reputable surgeons are comfortable with any "clear margin". It's a matter of individual preference and comfort When a lumpectomy specimen is removed, it may be marked by the surgeon as to its different sides so that if one side has too narrow a margin or a margin involved with cancer, the surgeon can go back and take more tissue to assure a negative margin. For most small tumors and even some large tumors, lumpectomy is becoming the standard of therapy.

In many instances, lumpectomy is accompanied by sentinel node (*see* chapter on Sentinel Node Dissection) or axillary lymph node dissection.

Axillary Lymph Node Dissection

When you have been told you need to have an axillary lymph node dissection, this means that the surgeon will be removing the lymph nodes in the armpit that lie generally just below the axillary vein. To remove these, the surgeon must also remove the fatty tissue in which they are enveloped, and this will create a hollow area and moderate deformity. Unless this procedure is done in conjunction with a mastectomy, a separate incision is made in the axilla as shown (figure 25) and the tissue is removed using sharp (knife and scissors) or blunt (grasping and pulling or teasing) dissection. Bleeding is controlled by cautery, little titanium clips on the blood vessels (Hemoclips) or ties and suture (thread and needle).

When the dissection is completed, the surgeon must leave two motor nerves (nerves that effect motion of a muscle), the long thoracic nerve (which supplies the chest wall muscle called the serratus), and the thoracodorsal nerve (which innervates the big latissimus muscle, the "lats"). Injury to the long thoracic nerve may cause weakness of the muscle that holds your shoulder blade or scapula against your back, and you get a "winged scapula". If the nerve is injured and not cut, normal function usually returns in a few weeks. Injury to the other nerve, the thoracodorsal, is less serious and causes some weakness and tiredness of the arm motion at the shoulder. Injury to the first intercostal or intercostobrachial sensory (feeling only--not motion) nerve will leave an area of numbness at the back of the axilla and in a portion of the upper arm as shown. Frequently, division of this nerve is necessary to complete the axillary dissection, and it is often "taken" by surgeons. (*See* chapter on Complications). Most surgeons place a tube drain in the axilla after doing a lymph node dissection, and it should remain in place for several days or until the drainage becomes minimal.

To prevent the complication of lymphedema (swelling of the arm), all my patients are referred to physical therapists who instruct them on exercise and lymphedema prevention, and give them the necessary education to prevent any major post-operative axillary complications. (*See* Lymphedema chapter).

Modified Radical Mastectomy

When do we need to do a modified radical mastectomy? Remember that in most cases, when we do a lumpectomy, we need to follow this with radiation to the remaining breast to lower the high incidence of locally recurrent breast cancer. Some individuals refuse to have radiation because of the time required for treatment, or they may have had previous radiation to that breast, and cannot receive more radiation. Still others who have a diagnosis of cancer may want to have the breast removed for emotional reasons. This operation consists of removal of all the breast tissue along with the nipple-areolar complex, and doing the above described axillary dissection. The large muscles on the anterior chest wall are preserved. The incision for this surgery is quite variable but is usually some type of ellipse around the front of the breast including the nipple and areola, and extending towards the axilla. When all the tissue is removed, one or two drains are placed, and the skin is closed with either under-the--skin absorbable sutures, nylon sutures or staples, and steri-strip (paper band-aid) dressings are applied along with a bulky gauze and circumferential wrap. Patients usually stay overnight, and are sent home the next day with drains in place.

Some women opt for immediate breast reconstruction, and for these, a plastic surgeon will give them information prior to the operation. After the breast surgeon has completed the mastectomy, the plastic surgeon takes over to do one of his reconstructions which may be placement of an "expander", a "TRAM or latissimus flap" or in a rare case, actual placement of an implant. (*See* Plastic Surgery chapter).

Radical Mastectomy

This procedure, the operation described by Dr. William Halsted in the 1890's, was the surgery of choice for breast cancer for almost 60 years. Today it is rarely used because it has been replaced by the modified radical mastectomy. This operation differs from the modified procedure in that the surgeon removes the large chest wall muscles, the pectoralis major and pectoralis minor, and often takes so much skin that a primary closure is not possible, and a skin graft is needed to cover the opening. It is a very deforming operation, and even plastic reconstruction is more difficult and less satisfactory. The only real indications today are when a cancer invades the muscles, and no other recourse will allow complete removal of the tumor. In the past, "super-radical" operations were also done, but are no longer recommended, and don't need to be described to you.

Simple, Subcutaneous and Skin-Sparing Mastectomies

These are essentially procedures where most or all of the breast tissue is removed.

The simple mastectomy is a modified radical mastectomy without an axillary node dissection. The nipple and areola are taken out as in that operation. This type of procedure is done on a woman who has had a prior lumpectomy and axillary dissection who comes up with a recurrence or new tumor in the same breast, and the Cancer Committee decides that a mastectomy should be performed. The axillary nodes have already been removed.

The skin sparing mastectomy is performed through a smaller incision usually encompassing the nipple and areola, leaving most of the skin of the breast and allowing for a more natural reconstruction by the plastic surgeon. It takes more time and a special skill to complete this procedure through this "keyhole" type incision, but in skilled hands, it is just as effective as the simple mastectomy.

The subcutaneous mastectomy removes most of the breast tissue but leaves the nipple and areola. It is probably not an adequate cancer operation because much more breast tissue is left than I consider acceptable for a curative or preventative operation. It is, however, a good operation for benign disease. For example, in women with severe fibrocystic disease and painful breasts, where one desires to remove most of the symptomatic breast tissue and allow for a good reconstruction, this is an excellent operation, and is usually done well by the plastic surgeons.

Patients who have undergone surgical procedures for cancer in our hospital receive a discharge packet. (*See* Joanne O'Heany's chapter on the Information Center). This includes general information about Breast Cancer, Reach To Recovery, The Wig Bank, The Look Good, Feel Better Program, The Psychosocial Support Groups, the Lymphedema Program, and numerous informational pamphlets from the American Cancer Society. The patient goes home with the beginnings of a strong support group and with her questions, for the most part, answered. She is informed that her case will be reviewed at the next Breast Tumor Board by a panel of specialists, and that her physician and surgeon will discuss the findings and recommendations with her. Having undergone a very emotionally and often physically traumatic experience, she leaves the hospital with understanding, confidence and reassurance that she is being taken care of in a comprehensive manner at a highly sophisticated center of excellence.

Table I
PRE-OPERATIVE WORKUP
Preoperative Workup For Most Breast Surgery

CBC (Complete Blood Count)
Urinalysis
Electrolytes (in women over 40) measures body chemistry of Na (sodium), K (potassium), Cl (chlorides), CO_2 (carbon dioxide)
Chest X-ray (in women over 40 or if otherwise indicated)
EKG (Electrocardiogram—measuring heart function)
    in women over 40
UCG (Pregnancy Test) unless post-hysterectomy or post-menopausal

Other tests in special circumstances which your doctor may order:
    PT, PTT, INR—measures blood clotting ability
    Liver panel (SGOT, SPGT, LDH, bilirubin, alkaline phosphatase)
    if there is any question about liver disease or gallbladder disease

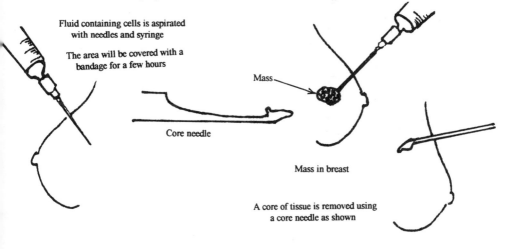

Fluid containing cells is aspirated with needles and syringe

The area will be covered with a bandage for a few hours

Mass

Core needle

Mass in breast

A core of tissue is removed using a core needle as shown

Figure 18. FINE NEEDLE ASPIRATION AND
STEREOTACTIC CORE BIOPSY.

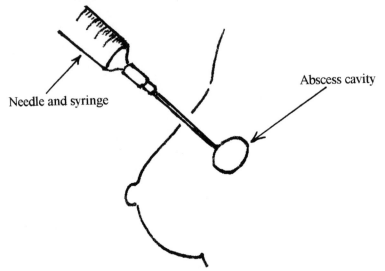

Needle and syringe

Abscess cavity

Figure 19. DRAINAGE OF AN ABSCESS.

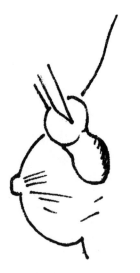

The lump is removed through a small incision

Figure 20. EXCISION OF A FIBROADENOMA.

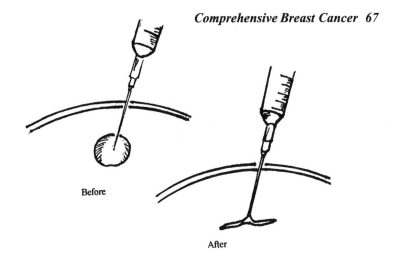

Before

After

Figure 21. ASPIRATION OF A CYST.

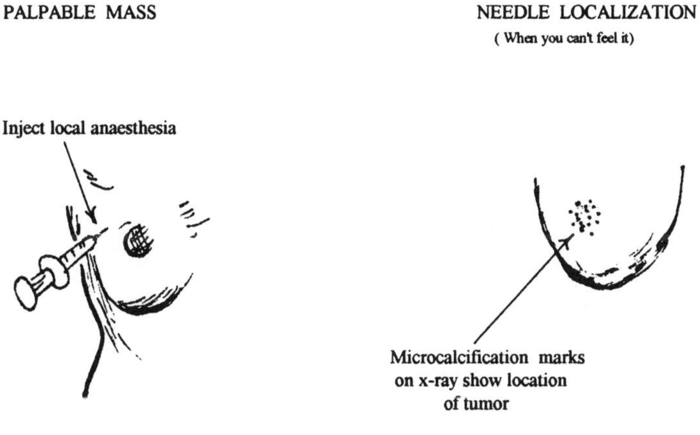

PALPABLE MASS

NEEDLE LOCALIZATION
(When you can't feel it)

Inject local anaesthesia

Microcalcification marks
on x-ray show location
of tumor

Figure 22. SIMPLE BIOPSY.

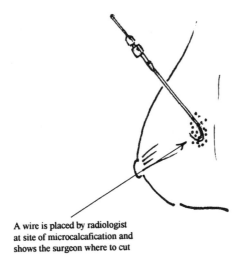

A wire is placed by radiologist
at site of microcalcafication and
shows the surgeon where to cut

Figure 23a. NEEDLE LOCALIZATION.

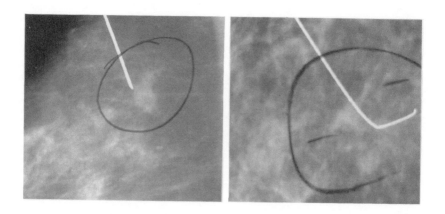

Figure 23b. NEEDLE LOCALIZATION.

LUMPECTOMY - NARROW, WIDE AND INVOLVED MARGINS

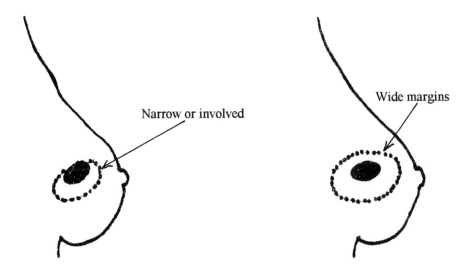

Figure 24. LUMPECTOMY.

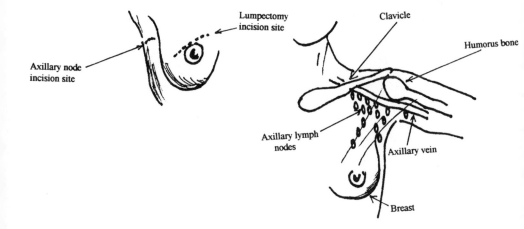

Figure 25. AXILLARY NODE DISSECTION.

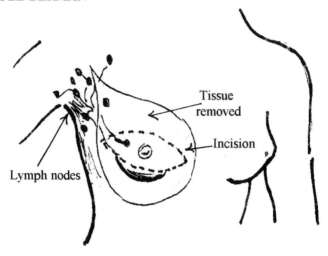

In a modified radical mastectomy, the surgeon removes
the breast and the lymph nodes under the arm.

Figure 26. MODIFIED RADICAL MASTECTOMY.

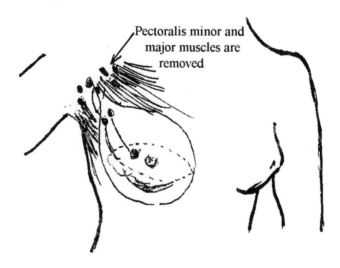

In a radical mastectomy the procedure is the same as the modified,
except the pectoralis minor and major muscles are removed

Figure 27. RADICAL MASTECTOMY.

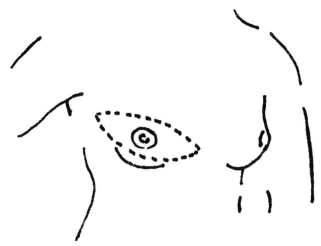

In total (simple) mastectomy, only the breast and
areola tissue is removed. The lymph nodes, most
of the skin and muscles are left in place.

Figure 28. SIMPLE MASTECTOMY.

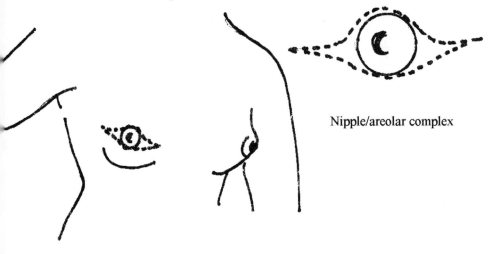

Nipple/areolar complex

...n sparing mastectomy there is a peri areolar incision,
...ving the nipple and areola, but leaving most of the skin.

Figure 29. SKIN SPARING MASTECTOMY.

Chapter 7
COMPLICATIONS
OF SURGERY

I've almost reached perfection, it's nearly in my grasp,
My halo's almost sitting right, it almost makes me gasp.
I'm oh so skilled at surgery, I'm smart, clever and brave
But I was told I won't be perfect 'till I'm in the grave.

And if I've not achieved perfection, that means I could fail,
Like sailing on a wind tossed sea with a slightly damaged sail.
My training was the best, I'm sure, and I've sailed there before,
But if the wind dies down I may be sailing with an oar.

To operate requires a skill and practice to do well,
But humans, like the tossing seas, occasionally rebel.
And the best laid plans of surgeons, sometimes go astray
And patients need to understand and put their ire away.

The surgeon without complications, never held a knife,
There is no perfect husband and there is no perfect wife.
The able sailors are the ones who recognize this fact
And know the steps to take to safely bring the frigate back.

Anyone can do a case when nothing at all goes wrong,
But only the ablest can correct a problem as it comes along.
Cutting into human flesh is not like changing a muffler
Surgery is less exact and is often a whole lot toughler.

L et's face it, as near to perfection as most surgeons think they are, they unfortunately have complications. And we must understand that complications fall into three categories: One, due to the incompetence of the surgeon; secondly due to patient behavior; and thirdly (and most common) due to the fact that people are not machines, and situations have a myriad of variables that may account for something not going the way we want it to.

The first problem, namely the incompetence of the surgeon, is one which can only be prevented by being careful and selective from the outset. Be sure your surgeon has the training and experience for the job before letting him practice on you Check his credentials and Board Certification, and know that he has done the surgery before, and that he is willing to work in a milieu such as we have described in the Comprehensive Breast Care Management discussion. And remember that no surgeon is perfect, and that sometimes errors can occur by the most prominent, well-trained, and experienced hands. That does not constitute incompetence; it underlines the fact that we are all human.

The second issue concerns you, the patient. When you place yourself in the hands of a surgeon, you need to understand his requirements for you as a patient. I have the greatest difficulty when treating other physicians because they don't know how to be patients; they don't take direction well in the pre- and postoperative periods, and usually end up with complications that are usually avoided by the compliant patient. If you become too controlling and directive, you will hinder your surgeon's ability to practice the kind of medicine which he does well, and you will occasionally suffer for it. If you can't be comfortable or place your confidence and trust in your surgeon, step back, look to yourself, and probably get another surgeon. It's best for both of you.

So that leaves us with the third category: Complications occurring because we are humans and not machines--the so-called "Acts-of--God" reasons. And when you develop a complication, which probably bothers your surgeon almost as much as it bothers you (being perfectionists, surgeons generally have a hard time dealing with any type of failure or even partial failure!), remember that the worse thing to do in a difficult situation is to start accusing, pointing fingers of blame and getting unduly angry. If something happens, help the surgeon work to correct and resolve it. Obviously if something has been grossly mismanaged, your friendly attorney will be able to advise you adequately.

So what are the complications that can occur when you go in for breast surgery? The problems that accompany cosmetic procedures are best discussed by the plastic surgeon, and these doctors usually outline all the potential problems very carefully since the surgery is completely elective and cosmetic. In the procedures of augmentation and reduction mammoplasty, the problems include hematomas, seromas, sensation loss, occasional skin loss, sloughing of the nipple and areola, size differences, infection, and movement of the implant into an unacceptable position, or "hardening" of the implant. ("I wanted them bigger" won't hold water!) These conditions are all correctable with further procedures, and occasionally grafting of skin, and removal and replacement of an implant is necessary. In major reconstructions such as those described in the Plastic Surgery chapter, TRAM and latissimus flaps may not survive, or there may be partial loss of skin or subcutaneous tissue. Enough for plastic surgery. Let's get to the basic breast surgery, and the things that can occur in the best of hands.

Biopsies of the breast, whether needle, core or open, can always result in delayed bleeding which can cause the subcutaneous tissue and skin to "stain" with blood (which may turn from red to yellow to normal, much like a "black eye"), and if the bleeding occurs deep inside the breast, it may result in a mass, or a collection of blood or serum. For the skin staining (ecchymosis), there is no real treatment except for ice compresses and observation to make sure it doesn't progress. For the deeper hematoma or seroma, the fluid can usually be aspirated painlessly in the office by a surgeon. When large fluid collections occur, a drain may need to be placed and left for several days. The resultant breast may have a "hard" area for several months, and a smaller area of firmness may persist for a long time. Only rarely will a hematoma require a more serious surgical intervention in the operating room, where the patient will need the wound opened, the bleeding site secured (that's a surgeon's euphemism for sewing it up!), and the wound reclosed, usually over a temporary drain. This is usually done under a general anesthetic but under some circumstances, can be done with sedation and a local anesthetic.

A patient may ask: "Why did I bleed?" to which the surgeon sheepishly but truthfully replies: "It was dry when I left". Basically, when blood vessels are cut during surgery, the body responds by causing the vessel to retract and for the muscles in the wall of the vessel to constrict, stopping the bleeding for a while. Under most conditions, the surgeon electrocoagulates bleeding vessels or ties them. But occasionally the vessel retracts and seals off without being seen. Several hours later, these vessels have usually "clotted off" on their own and when the muscle retraction reverses, even then there will be no bleeding. But occasionally the vessel doesn't stay constricted long enough or the "clot" isn't strong enough, and bleeding starts, much to the distress of the patient and the chagrin of the surgeon. To prevent this, I routinely wrap the breasts with a very snug Ace bandage after most procedures, and have been very satisfied with the results.

Biopsies and other surgeries can get infected, and usually respond to antibiotics. However, if the deep tissue is severely infected, then an abscess (a collection of pus) may occur, and the patient needs to have this drained either in the physician's office, or if very severe, in the operating room. I used to try and do many procedures in the office but now feel more comfortable doing them in the operating room where conditions are optimal. Surgeons should handle any complication in the best possible manner, and shouldn't be afraid or ashamed to have to "take the patient back to the operating room".

Surgeons differ in their method of wound closures, and occasionally the sutures themselves can cause problems. When self-absorbing sutures are used in skin closure, they usually dissolve in several weeks. In some people, these sutures (especially the little knots) may get infections or protrude through the skin, and they may need to be removed by the surgeon. When non-absorbable sutures are used, there may be differing degrees of skin reactions from mild to severe, requiring earlier-than-usual suture removal. These problems usually do not result in lasting problems. And you will know if you are a "scar former". Some individuals with the same exact closure techniques end up with almost invisible scars whereas others will have a raised, wide ugly reminder of their surgery (keloid). If you know that you are a "scar former", tell your surgeon, and he may inject the wound with a steroid compound which at least lessens the severity of the scar. And finally, remember that surgery involves opening the skin, and unless you're from planet X or know the surgeons who worked on The Six Million Dollar Man or Woman, there will be scars and some deformity, no matter how slight. They are usually coverable by cosmetics. Be realistic!

A more minor complication of any surgery is hematoma and small blood clots in the area where you have an IV needle. Although uncomfortable, they almost always resolve fairly rapidly with warm compresses.

Let's go on to the other surgical procedures. Lumpectomy is usually very straight forward but the same complications that occur during a simple open biopsy can occur in this procedure. Just think of a lumpectomy as an extended biopsy--more incision, more tissue removed, more chances of complication, and slightly more severity. Similarly with mastectomy, except that in this case, the deformity is more severe, and we have to deal with the possible complication that the skin edges may be deprived of their blood supply (especially near the closure line), and may slough (another surgical euphemism for "die"--we don't like to use that word!). In case this occurs, there is usually enough skin to allow the surgeon to remove the dead tissue and reclose the wound, but occasionally a skin graft may be needed.

Now let us get to the major area of problem occurrence, the axilla. In addition to all the same problems found with breast biopsy, axillary dissection is fraught with many potential problems, and we try to anticipate them in the pre- and postoperative periods. We know that we are leaving a large "dead space" (a cavity remaining after a procedure which the body may try to fill with serum), and that seromas or blood collections may occur. For this reason we usually place drains for a short period of time, and wrap the patients with a snug Ace bandage as I have described before. Even still, after the drains are removed, hematomas and seromas can occur, which can either be aspirated by the surgeon in his office or require a replacement of the drain for a longer period of time.

I have described the various nerves of the axilla in the section on Anatomy, and will review the effects of damage or transection (complete cutting) of these nerves. The sensory nerve (intercostobrachial) supplies feeling to the back of the armpit and the first part of the upper inner arm. Sometimes this nerve is divided intentionally or accidentally during the dissection, and will cause numbness or a strange sensation in these areas. Although there will be some return of sensation, it's probably going to be permanent, but it is usually not a major or even a significantly minor problem. It cannot easily be repaired and probably should not be corrected because of the minimal nature of the problem.

The motor nerves (responsible for movement of muscles--*see* Anatomy) are an entirely different story. Unless they are extensively involved in tumor or scar tissue and avoiding their injury is not possible, they should always be preserved. I myself have never encountered a situation necessitating this procedure, but it can occur, and the surgeon must use his best judgment in these situations. The "winging" of the scapula occurs when the long thoracic nerve is cut (it supplies the muscle that holds the shoulder blade against the back). Sometimes the injury is only due to nerve damage and not complete division, and in these cases, the winged scapula will improve with time. However, the completely cut nerve results in permanent disability which, if desired, can only be corrected by an orthopedic surgical procedure. The thoracodorsal nerve, if cut, will cause a weakness and tiredness of the arm around the shoulder movement, and it should not be tremendously disabling unless you are an avid sportswoman--ie., playing golf, softball, bowling. I have never seen an injury to this nerve although it has been described.

There will be a hollowed out appearance to the armpit area of surgery, but its cosmetic appearance varies from individual to individual depending on body size, fat content, and the amount of tissue removed. Each surgeon does the dissection a little differently, and may get slightly different cosmetic results. Injury to the big vein in the axilla or injury to the large nerve bundles (the brachial plexus) supplying motor and sensory function to the arm and hand are so rare that they need not be discussed.

The last and yet definitely greatest complication of axillary node dissection is LYMPHEDEMA, and I consider it such a major problem that I have devoted an entire chapter to its description, attempts at prevention and treatment. It is a major problem which has, until recently, only been paid "lip-service" by surgeons, and yet it is the most major complaint of recovering breast cancer patients in group meetings.

Let us move on now to the last areas for discussion of complications, namely mastectomies. The modified radical, skin sparing, and simple mastectomies have all the same potential for complications as the lumpectomy with the addition of problems with the "skin flap" healing, possible wound separation, and severe cosmetic deformity. The latter is not really a complication but an expected after-effect of the surgery, and shouldn't be considered in this discussion. Wound healing problems may result from removing sutures too soon or because the patient has an underlying medical problem which makes for poor healing, such as diabetes mellitus, history of treatment with steroids, vascular (blood vessel) diseases affecting the skin (such as vasculitis, lupus erythematosus, polyarteritis), previous radiation therapy, infection or injury to the surgical site (ie., blunt trauma by a kicking baby). Wound separations can usually be closed without much setback in the healing process, but when they are complex, the plastic surgeon may be called in for consultation and assistance.

Patients requiring the old radical mastectomy have the large pectoralis major and smaller pectoralis minor muscles removed as part of the procedure. Reconstruction by the plastic surgeon is more difficult and is less cosmetically satisfying, and the absence of the muscles leads to more significant weakness of the arm, and some limitation of movement around the shoulder. When a large area of skin is removed, a primary (edge to edge) closure of the wound may not be possible, and skin grafting or rotation flaps (*see* Plastic Surgery) may be necessary.

In conclusion, let's just say that breast surgery, although on the surface of the body, (not for example in the chest or abdominal cavities or involving major surgery on blood vessels or nerves) may still have all the various complications of a major surgery. These are scary to consider but they occur so rarely that to focus on them to any great degree is unwarranted. These include pulmonary emboli (blood clots going to the lung), heart and lung problems, and bizarre, rare anesthetic problems. Whereas years ago all patients remained in bed for days after any surgery, most of today's breast surgery patients are ambulated (encouraged to get up and walk) as soon as possible after the anesthetic wears off, and many procedures are done on an outpatient basis. This prevents many of the old complications caused by inactivity including the pulmonary embolism, pneumonia, and developing stiff muscles around the "shoulder girdle" (the muscles and bony structures of the shoulder).

Chapter 8
SENTINEL NODE BIOPSY

I found out that I am a sentinel node
(I didn't just know it), I was recently told.
I'm radioactive and also I'm blue,
The doctors all say that I'm something quite new.
If I'm not lined with cancer when under detection
They don't have to do a wide lymph node dissection.

In previous sections, we have talked about the axillary lymph node dissection accompanying lumpectomy, and as a part of the standard modified radical mastectomy. The Comprehensive Breast Team uses the information obtained from these lymph nodes to determine a plan of further treatment for the patient with breast cancer. There has been a steady movement away from the more radical breast surgical procedures, as from the radical mastectomy to the modified radical mastectomy to the lumpectomy, but all of these have required the surgeon to do a dissection in the axilla, removing the lymph nodes, and evaluating for the presence or absence of metastatic cancer. We have discussed the complications of axillary lymph node dissection, and emphasized in a separate chapter the problems and management of lymphedema.

A new approach to the problem has been the Sentinel Lymph Node theory. We now believe that the drainage of lymph or debris from each area of the breast follows a very orderly pattern as seen in the diagram. We feel that in this orderly flow, there is one or more first set of lymph nodes which we will call the Sentinel Nodes (a sentinel is a guard or a warning of danger), and I guess the person who coined the words meant it as a warning or signal node. The theory is that a cancer of the breast will go first to the sentinel node draining that area of the breast. Those who support this theory propose that if a sentinel node does not have cancer in it, then the rest of the lymph nodes in the axilla are cancer-free. Initially, reports were very supportive of this theory, and false negatives were extremely rare (a situation where the sentinel node is negative but the axillary nodes were positive for cancer). And if this is so, then the sentinel node can indeed be a predictor of the axillary nodes. The opposite, of course, would be that if the sentinel node is positive for tumor cells, then there is a very strong possibility that there are further positive nodes in the axilla. Unfortunately, there is additional data in the medical literature now to challenge this hypothesis, and the final answers are not yet out. Suffice it to say, this theory probably holds true for the most part in what we have called Stage I breast cancers and can be used safely in these cases.

So how do we identify these sentinel nodes, and how does this effect our surgical procedures and our outcomes?

The sentinel nodes can be identified in two distinct ways: The first is by injecting a special blue dye into the area of the cancer and waiting a short while (10 to 20 minutes), gently massaging the breast. When making a small incision in the upper outer area of the breast, the surgeon can usually see the blue streaks of dye in the lymphatic channels leading toward a little lymph node or a group of lymph nodes. These are called the sentinel nodes. A second method is called lymphoscintigraphy. This is a fancy word encompassing the injection of a weak radioactive liquid into the area of the tumor, and having the patient lie under a special scanning machine that traces the flow of the nucleotide (radioactive liquid) along the lymphatic channels towards and into the axilla. The first area where it accumulates is understood to be the location of the sentinel nodes. A picture is taken of this "lymph node mapping" by the nuclear medicine technologist, and the location of the node is marked on the patient's body. The patient then goes to surgery, and the surgeon uses a hand-held "counter" (like a Geiger Counter) to further localize the area of radioactivity, and thereby identify the sentinel node. Many physicians use both methods to act as a control, and check and to make identification easier.

This type of sentinel node "biopsy" takes practice (up to 30 trials are recommended before becoming proficient), and only the surgeon who has practiced should rely on this procedure alone without doing the full axillary dissection. In many centers, the sentinel node dissection is routinely done on low grade cancers, and if the node is negative, they do not go ahead with the axillary lymph node dissection. Ask your own surgeon about this as it will be up to his judgment whether he considers the procedure safe and accurate.

Suffice it to say, if you can get by without the axillary node dissection, you will not have to face the many complications found with that procedure including hematoma, seroma, nerve and muscle damage and most of all, the potential for lymphedema (*see* Lymphedema chapter).

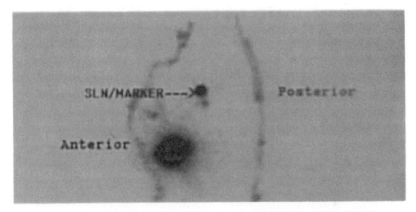

Figure 30. A PHOTOGRAPH OF LYMPHOSCINTIGRAPHY.

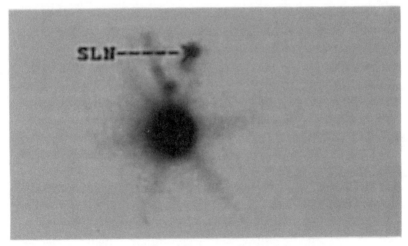

Figure 31. SENTINEL LYMPH NODE (SLN).

Chapter 9
LYMPHEDEMA
AND MANAGEMENT OF COMPLICATIONS OF AXILLARY DISSECTION FROM A PHYSICAL THERAPIST'S VIEWPOINT

Lymphedema's a problem we need to consider
It occurs sometimes after your nodes are removed.
A woman can sometimes become very bitter,
If it happens and nothing can make it improve.

So we give women lessons on how to prevent
This occurrence with physical therapy training,
And having the courage to never relent,
The problem's not solved, but we're certainly gaining.

It can happen tomorrow or in several years.
You'll be taught arm massage and avoid all abuses,
And hopefully we can allay all your fears
And your arm will stay supple and have all its uses.

But it does require care and an ounce of prevention
No heavy lifting, blood draws or blood pressure,
And if you are diligent, it remains our contention
The problem will slowly resolve in good measure.

L ymphedema is probably the most complained about complication occurring after axillary dissection alone, after axillary radiation therapy, and after the combination of the two. It is caused by a destruction of the normal lymphatic channels which drain lymph from your arm into the central part of your body when the lymph nodes under the arm are removed by a surgeon or destroyed by radiation therapy. We will focus on this problem as a *fait accompli* now, since we have discussed some of the newer surgery which is eliminating some of the need for axillary dissection, and therefore obviating this problem.

Because the surgeon does not have microscopic vision, he/she cannot see the extent to which the lymph nodes are being removed in the axilla and in the area of the axillary vein (*see* Anatomy), and so there is no easy way to assess how complete or destructive the surgery will be. The body is different from individual to individual and the lymphatic channels vary considerably. With similar surgical procedures, some women will have sufficient residual lymphatic channels to offset the possibility of a "lymph backup" and others may not. Some surgeons are actually changing their axillary node dissection techniques so as to leave more of the normal nodes in place around the vein and concentrate more on the nodes in the lower part of the armpit. But be sure to discuss this with your surgeon prior to surgery. The National Lymphedema Network has developed a pink wristband for patients after axillary dissection to remind caregivers not to start IV's, take blood pressure or draw blood from the involved arm. We shall talk more about prevention and treatment, but suffice it to say that awareness of the problem, its potential severity and if untreated, the progressive and irreversible damage that can be caused, cannot be overemphasized.

A few years ago at a medical conference I was talking with several colleagues and the subject of lymphedema came up. All of the surgeons present stated that they rarely ever saw a case and that they did not consider it a major problem. Several of the oncologists and a clinical psychologist were also present, and they laid to rest any doubts about the severity of the problem. The therapist stated that lymphedema was the single most major problem women spoke about in their support groups and one to which their surgeons paid only the slightest lip service. Similarly, the oncologists who would see the patients for years after the surgery was completed supported this view. The surgeons were very surprised and many went back to their practices to check on previous breast surgery patients, and found the incidence of lymphedema to be much higher than they expected. In September, 1998, I attended a conference on lymphedema organized by the National Lymphedema Network and the title of the conference was (and very appropriately so) "Lymphedema: Uncovering the Hidden Epidemic". Needless to say, the attendees were primarily physical therapists, several patients with lymphedema, and very few physicians. It is a problem which is just beginning to "come out of the closet".

Today, any comprehensive breast care center should have a lymphedema prevention and treatment program. This is one complication which must be anticipated and managed long before the earliest symptoms develop. If you wait for symptoms to occur, you may have missed the window of opportunity for prevention and optimal management. Surgeons must be educated and if it takes the patient to do the educating, then so be it. Remember to discuss this issue with your surgeon prior to any surgery involving the axilla and if need be, hook up with a local representative of the National Lymphedema Network for further advise and counseling.

Lymphedema may occur soon after surgery with or without radiation or may develop insidiously over several months or years. I have seen cases that developed more than ten years after a woman's definitive surgery, brought on by a small injury or infection in the arm.

What is the incidence of this complication? The medical literature varies tremendously but the generally accepted figures are about 8-10% of women after axillary node dissection, 8-12% after radiation alone, and up to 30% or more after combination axillary lymph node surgery and radiation. So it is a real and major problem.

Before we progress to lymphedema secondary to breast cancer treatment, I want to mention that there is a condition called Primary Lymphedema which a man or woman may develop from birth without any known etiology. We will not focus on this and will only be talking about Secondary Lymphedema or lymphedema acquired as a result of the surgery and/or radiation you have for treatment of breast cancer.

There are several stages of lymphedema but it is important to recognize the early warnings indicating that a problem may be developing. These are signs and symptoms which may be apparent before actual swelling of the arm is seen. These include pain or aching in the extremity, progressive numbness, and loss of normal mobility of the arm. There may be increased frequency of minor, poorly healing sores of the extremity (since the lymphatic system is not draining normally). These are the sentinel events that should tell you to be ever more alert for other problems and to work on the preventative and therapeutic measures we shall cover later in this chapter.

There are three stages of lymphedema. Stage I is "Pitting Edema"—a reversible situation when treated vigorously. (This is a condition where there is an accumulation of fluid in the extremity, and when the skin is touched or pushed, a "pit" or indentation occurs). The earliest sign may be a ring which is suddenly too tight or slight swelling of the arm, or that a small scratch too readily develops into an infection. These events have to be identified and treatment started as soon as possible. Frequently a woman, especially many years after breast cancer treatment, will downplay the seriousness of these warnings and put off seeing a physician or therapist expecting the condition to resolve spontaneously. It usually doesn't go away very quickly. So heed the warning signs and don't delay.

Stage II Lymphedema is characterized by protein-rich edema (thicker, less watery fluid) and progressive hardening of the extremity. This is more severe and not spontaneously reversible. The limb becomes very swollen and painful with a significant change in mobility and swelling of the hands and fingers which may make grasping and fine digital work impossible. Without careful monitoring and vigorous treatment, a person with the symptoms of Stage I lymphedema can progress to Stage II in a few months. But this is still treatable and much of the condition can be ameliorated if vigorous treatment is instituted. You may never get back to a "normal" or "pre-lymphedema" state, but most function can be returned and discomfort can be significantly diminished.

Since Stage I and Stage II will alter the appearance of your arm, this "disease" of lymphedema will strongly impact your emotional condition. It is "seen" at work and socializing and will affect the way you feel about yourself. It has been said that those who suffer from lymphedema suffer as much and sometimes more from the physical deformity as from the pain and other symptoms. So it's important to recognize and handle the skin problems at a very early stage. There are lymphedema support groups throughout the country to help in the psychosocial problems encountered by these women.

Unfortunately, because of the lack of awareness, there are situations where the condition is not recognized early and sadly women progress to Stage III lymphedema. This is an irreversible condition with chronic hardening of the skin (in the lower extremity, it's called elephantiasis since the limb is very large and firm), secondary to scarring and fibrosis occurring in all layers of the skin with recurring infections, pain and marked limitation of motion. In long term chronic lymphedema, a rare occurrence is a cancer of the lymphatic system called lymphangiosarcoma. Stage III lymphedema is treatable but not reversible and we will be discussing some of the methods for making patients more comfortable when they have this condition.

How do we diagnose this condition? There are no standard criteria for diagnosis but the knowledgeable physician in the comprehensive center should be able to identify the signs and symptoms at an early stage. It takes no great clinical acumen to make the diagnosis when a woman comes in with a big, swollen, painful arm Frequently the woman makes the diagnosis herself and asks her doctor what to do about it. There are some diagnostic procedures which can be used such as Doppler flow measurement (measuring blood flow in the arm), magnetic resonance imaging (MRI), and computer tomography (CAT scan) which will show changes in later stages of the disease. Lymphoscintigraphy (LAS) is a big word to describe injecting a minimally radioactive material into the involved arm and mapping out the lymphatic system. One can actually determine how severe the damage to the lymphatic system has been by evaluating this study and appropriate treatments can be designed. So let us now move on to prevention and treatment.

Every one of my patients undergoing any axillary surgery has a preoperative and postoperative consultation with a physical therapist trained in the prevention, management, and treatment of lymphedema so that no patient leaves the hospital without a handful of pamphlets and an earful of advice and recommendations. The following is the information from our lymphedema physical therapy specialist, Shari Fusco, P.T.

PHYSICAL THERAPY

Prior to undergoing surgery for breast cancer, whether it be for a mastectomy or a lumpectomy, the patient must be educated on the causes and prevention of Lymphedema. Any patient who has axillary lymph node dissection or undergoes radiation treatment is at risk for lymphedema. The patient is given a list of skin care precautions to prevent lymphedema (*see* Table). The patient needs to follow these precautions for the rest of her life because lymphedema can occur days, weeks, months, or many years after the breast cancer surgery has occurred.

Following mastectomy surgery, the patient is educated again on the risks and causes of lymphedema, and on the role of physical therapy in their recovery. The goal of physical therapy is for the patient to regain full range of motion and strength in the affected arm and to prevent lymphedema. Once the drain tubes are removed from the surgical site, the patient can begin to restore shoulder function. One complication of immobility is a "frozen shoulder", which is inflammation of the shoulder capsule. This can cause an even greater amount of pain and discomfort which can last for months. This is why it is important to start mobilizing the affected arm early after the surgery.

There are three complications or complaints that most women have after a mastectomy and/or axillary node dissection; one complication being hypersensitivity in the upper, inner affected arm and chest wall. Patients complain of sensations of burning tingling, and numbness. These surfaces are numb because the nerves in the skin that supply sensation were cut during the operation. These sensations are normal and their skin may be numb months to years after the surgery. There is no treatment for this hypersensitivity; you just have to wait for it to subside. This hypersensitivity often leads to a loss of shoulder range of motion, secondary to guarding the joint from any painful stimuli. This is often true when it is the non-dominant arm that is affected.

A second possible complication after axillary node dissection is the residual fold of skin under the arm where the lymph nodes were removed. The superficial lymphatic vessels have been damaged; therefore they become taut and shrink because they no longer carry lymphatic fluid. This residual fold can lead to a feeling of tightness, pain, and a decrease in shoulder range of motion. Most women have relief in pain when they continue to do the stretching exercises and skin mobilization. Modalities such as ultrasound can also be used for pain relief.

A third possible complication is that the pectoralis major muscle can cramp and have spasm. This often occurs when the patient guards the arm and does not perform the stretching and range of motion exercises. Therefore, it is important that the patient start to use the arm normally as soon as possible.

The patient is initially instructed in active, assertive range of motion and stretching exercises; the most important being to improve shoulder flexion for overhead reaching. The patient is taught to grasp the affected arm with the unaffected arm and raise it above the head. The patient is then instructed in side-arm stretching. Hold the wrist of the affected side with the unaffected side. Rest the hands on top of the head with elbows bent. Slowly pull the arm of the affected side toward the head trying to touch the arm to the ear. Wall climb stretch is also used to increase shoulder flexion. The patient faces the wall and begins to "walk" her fingers up the wall and then holds the stretch. These are just a few stretches that can be used to increase range of motion in the shoulder joint.

Ultrasound is a modality often used by physical therapists to increase blood flow and tissue repair to an area of the body. Ultrasound can be used to decrease pain and tightness under the affected arm where the lymphatic vessels have become tightened, secondary to lymph node dissection. By decreasing the patient's pain and tightness, they are better able to tolerate stretching exercises to increase their shoulder range of motion. A person should not have ultrasound treatment if they have lymphedema, cellulitis, or a tendency to form blood clots in the arm. Ultrasound should never be used over an area where there is a known or suspected metastasis of tumor.

Skin mobilization is another important aspect in increasing mobility in the affected arm. There is a restriction of the skin under the arm and less skin on the chest where the breast was removed, making it more painful and difficult to move the arm. The patient is taught how to perform slow circular motions along the incision with their fingers to loosen the scar tissue that has formed in the area. This is often done in front of the mirror after a warm shower. The heat helps to soften the skin and make it easier for the fingers to glide across the skin.

There is a significant risk of lymphedema occurring following a mastectomy or lumpectomy secondary to axillary node dissection. If any of the following signs and/or symptoms occur such as redness, swelling, warmth to touch, or tenderness, the patient should contact their physician immediately. It is then the responsibility of the physician to refer the patient to a certified lymphedema program.

A certified lymphedema therapist will initially assess the patient's range of motion, strength, and swelling in the affected arm. The therapist will then develop an individual treatment plan that will enable the patient to achieve maximum function of the affected arm. The treatment approach most commonly used is Complete Decongestive Physiotherapy, which consists of compression machines, manual lymph drainage, bandaging, exercise, skin care, and patient education.

A compression machine is a sequential pump that forces compressed air through a multi-chamber sleeve that fits over the entire length of the arm. The theory is that this compression will move the edema out of the limb into the chest. However, it does not remove the protein from the tissue, which can become fibrotic and further impede lymphatic flow. This treatment is typically done in the physical therapy office and lasts from two to ten hours, depending on the amount of edema in the arm. Contraindications for use of the compression pump are: Primary lymphedema, blood vessel disease, metastatic cancer in affected limb, massive edema secondary to congestive heart failure, gangrene, dermatitis, deep venous thrombosis, and cellulitis.

Manual lymph drainage (MLD) is a massage technique of gentle stroking of the skin. It is designed to open up the lymphatic system in the affected limb and trunk as a means to remove the lymphatic fluid. It is a gentle massage because the lymphatic vessels are superficial and can be damaged with a forceful massage, unless there is scar tissue formation in a particular area. This treatment is done daily for two to four weeks.

Manual lymph drainage is then followed by a sequence of bandaging on the affected arm. The bandage consists of three layers and must be worn 24 hours a day, except when showering. The first layer is gauze, which is wrapped around individual fingers and then up the arm. The second layer is padding for compression. The third layer is a low stretch bandage. Once the circumference of the arm has stabilized, the patient is fitted for an elastic compression sleeve to maintain progress. This sleeve must be worn continuously for several months, and then can gradually be decreased if the arm remains stable. Compression sleeve should never be worn if there are signs of infection such as redness, warmth, open wounds, or increased inflammation.

The therapist will teach the patient and/or caregiver how to perform massage techniques; bandaging, compression garment application, and exercises, in order to maintain the progress made with the therapy. The therapist will design an exercise regimen to maintain and/or increase range of motion, and improve lymphatic flow in the affected arm.

It is important that if someone has lymphedema that they follow these guidelines:

(1) Avoid lifting heavy objects.
(2) Avoid vigorous repetitive movements against resistance.
(3) Continue exercise program to prevent loss of range of motion.
(4) Decrease weight to prevent further swelling.
(5) Wear compression garments in airplanes since changes in atmosphere can increase swelling.

The role of the physical therapist or certified lymphedema therapist is to educate the patient before and after a mastectomy, or removal of axillary lymph nodes, in the prevention of lymphedema, and how to restore normal movement in the affected arm. If lymphedema does occur, it is the responsibility of the therapist to educate the patient and develop a treatment program consisting of Complete Decongestive Physiotherapy.

STAGES OF LYMPHEDEMA

Stage I   Pitting Edema - Reversible when treated vigorously.

Stage II   Protein Rich Edema - Progressive hardening of extremity - more severe - not spontaneously reversible, hands and fingers very swollen and painful, transient partial loss of function. Treatable and significantly reversible.

Stage III   Irreversible hardening of skin secondary to scarring and fibrosis with recurring infection, pain and limitation of motion. Treatable but not reversible.

CAUSES OF LYMPHEDEMA IN BREAST DISEASE

Axillary Lymph Node Dissection
Axillary Radiation
Combination Axillary Lymph Node Dissection plus Radiation

TREATMENT OF LYMPHEDEMA STAGE I

Decongestive Therapy

Manual Lymph Drainage (MLD) as part of Complete Decongestive Physiotherapy (CDP)

Massage by lymphedema therapist

Wrapping with bandages

Avoidance of additional damage:
Certain sports
Compression by jewelry
Injuries
Lifting and extremity exercise
Extremes heat or cold
Blood pressure measurement
Blood draws

TREATMENT OF LYMPHEDEMA STAGE II

Same as Stage One plus

More Vigorous Decongestive Therapy Including
1. Careful skin cleansing and lubrication
2. Manual pressure to move fluid and redirect lymphatic flow.
3. Appropriate wrapping.
4. Individual exercise programs.

Chronic Use of Compression garments.

Other treatments available:
Antibiotics
Steroids
Benzopyrones
Diuretics
Surgery

Alternative Methods of Questionable Effectiveness:
Acupuncture
Hypnotherapy
Guided Imagery
Herbal Medicine
Meditation
Homeopathy

TREATMENT OF LYMPHEDEMA STAGE III

Same as Stage I and II
With poorer results!

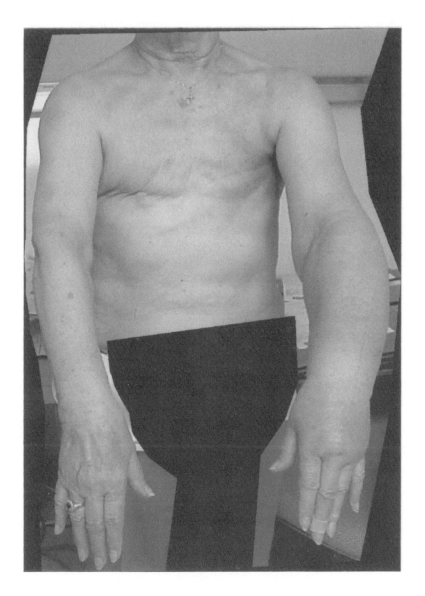

Figure 32. SEVERE LYMPHEDEMA AFTER
BILATERAL MASTECTOMY.

SKIN CARE PRECAUTIONS TO PREVENT LYMPHEDEMA

- Do not have blood pressure taken on the affected arm
- Never have injections or blood drawn in the affected arm
- Wearleather gloves and long sleeve shirts when working in the garden
- Avoid cat scratches
- Wear rubber gloves when cleaning to avoid skin irritation and minor injuries
- Protect yourself from insect bites with repellent and long sleeve shirt
- Use an electric razor, instead of a blade, when saving under the arm
- Take good care of your fingernails and cuticles
- Avoid wearing tight fitting clothing and jewelry on the arm
- Use caution to avoid extreme changes in temperature, protect from sunburn and burns while cooking and bathing
- Weight control-reduce or eliminate salt (salt causes fluid retention) and fat (holds fluid in arm) from diet
- Avoid lifting heavy objects (limit to 15 lbs) and vigorous, repetitive movements
- Recommended exercises are walking, swimming, cycling, light aerobics
- Keep arm elevated above the heart when lying down
- Keep affected arm very clean, and inspect skin daily for any signs of infection
- Signs of infection: Redness of skin, skin feels warm to touch, swelling, marked tenderness, fever. You need to contact your doctor right away
- If a small wound occurs, clean with a mild soap and water. Apply hydrogen peroxide as an antiseptic. Apply topical antibacterial ointment and cover with a bandage. Monitor wound daily for signs and symptoms of infection and clean if bandage becomes wet or soiled.

Chapter 10
SECOND OPINION

A second opinion is what I want to do,
My doctor has green eyes and I want one with blue;
He's Asian and Jewish and his skin is quite brown
I want an albino who's from out of town.

I want one from Harvard or Princeton or Yale
And I want one who's giving advice that's on sale;
My doctor plays Mozart, I really don't dig it;
And besides I'm convinced that he's really a bigot.

So, for a second opinion, please give me a name
I'll make him quite happy, he won't be the same.
I'll send him a list of my friends and relations
As long as he's not from some poor third world nation.

I'm basically looking for someone with knowledge
I'd prefer a physician that went through a college.
And if he drives a foreign made car.
I 'm afraid he won't do, we won't get very far.

So please get me a specialist who can tell me good news
My old doctor's crazy and gives me the blues.
Today's new physicians look too young to treat me
And the old ones look ready to die when they meet me.

Damn doctors, I just want a second opinion
I don't want to join in a radical minion,
I think that I better just see Aunt Louise,
She probably knows more about every disease.

When faced with difficult problems, complications or unexpected results, patients often seek a second opinion. Most physicians welcome this request in an effort to reassure the patient and to allay any fears about their standard of care. As I have mentioned before, cancer treatment is no longer a "one physician" job, and specialists rely upon other specialists for advice, discussion of difficult problems, and just plain reassurance, especially when a "case" is not going well or some unusual circumstance has arisen. So let us, as physicians, look upon second opinions as something to be welcomed and not feared or shunned. Similarly, the patient should try to seek out advice in a manner which lets her physician understand that it is not necessarily his competence or decisions she is questioning, but a needed reinforcement for her in a time of great stress and occasionally confusion. When a physician tells a patient something she does not want to hear, it is sometimes natural to go to someone else in an attempt to hear a different answer, perhaps the one which was sought after in the first place. And there are often patients who go from physician to physician, seeking out someone who will validate her thoughts and opinions, and treat her in the manner she wants rather than in the manner which medical prudence dictates. As seen in the chapter of Complementary and Alternative Therapies, sometimes patients seek completely nonvalid treatments, and miss the opportunity for help from a legitimate physician.

But let us consider the individual who wants a second opinion from a reputable source. Where does she go? First of all, she needs to evaluate the credentials of the group or the doctor she is seeking. Not so easy as it may seem. Anyone with a medical license can hang a shingle and claim to be an expert in this or that. Let me give you an example. The whole field of plastic and reconstructive surgery is rife with individuals claiming to be cosmetic surgeons, and yet many of them are not adequately trained or credentialed. Few people realize that Plastic Surgeons can be board certified by the American Board of Plastic Surgery, and that these are surgeons specially trained, for example, to do cosmetic breast surgery such as augmentation mammoplasties (implants), reduction mammoplasties, and breast reconstructions. And yet, because this type of surgery is often "paid up front" and financially lucrative, other physicians, not plastic surgeons, label themselves as "cosmetic surgeons", and do quite well attracting clientele to their offices. A general surgeon, an ENT (Ear Nose and Throat) or Eye (ophthalmologist) physician or even a general practitioner practicing out of his office, may be able to do breast "implants" if he wishes, without control from the state. Suffice it to say, when seeking out plastic and reconstructive surgery, a woman should look at the physician's credentials carefully, and not believe everything she sees. Each specialty and subspecialty usually has a National Board to which a physician trained in that specialty may apply. If he or she becomes a Diplomate of that board (passes their tests), it indicates that his peers consider the individual qualified to do the work of that specialty. Sure there are some exceptions, and some well qualified physicians may not be board certified, but it is at least a good guideline to follow. Also remember that there are many specialty boards but usually only one in each specialty which has validity. You might question why a surgeon doing augmentation mammoplasties would only be certified by the American Board of Cosmetic Surgery rather than the official American Board of Plastic and Reconstructive Surgery...I won't comment further on this. Similarly, when seeking treatment or second opinions, make sure that the physician, whether a general surgeon, radiation therapist, oncologist, etc., is appropriately trained in that specialty, and hopefully board certified by that specialty!

When going for a second opinion, you may have to spend some money outside what your health insurance will cover, but it may be well worth the expense to you both medically and emotionally. You may well go back to your original physician realizing that he's as great a physician as you first thought Also, don't just use outside information and the computer "net" as your sole second opinion. I can assure you that very little in the field of breast health is so cut and dry that you can get final answers from a book or a computer readout. I go to many meetings each year, and converse with other physicians daily to resolve the many issues that arise in my medical practice, and I am sure that its not easy for a nonmedical person to get a good understanding of an issue such as breast cancer, without direct interaction with a trained physician. Beware of "inexpert expert advice" from the popular magazines, newspapers, your next door neighbor or aunt Tillie.

And let me conclude by saying that most major medical centers and hopefully the major comprehensive breast centers have second opinion programs. There is usually a panel of physicians who can be consulted about certain matters and, in cases of cancer, usually a "tumor board" where cases can be presented for general discussion and advice (*see* chapter of "The Tumor Board"). When you have questions about your disease and your care that aren't answered to your satisfaction by your physician, before you seek out a second opinion, sit down with your physician and tell him about your concerns. Sometimes I am not even aware that a patient has certain questions about her care until I have had a second "sit-down discussion" with her. Remember that although a patient has access to excellent information on the Internet, this knowledge is not always tempered with the experience of a physician with the patient's individual concerns.

And finally, no matter how I, as a physician, behave with my patients, there is always occasionally a situation where the doctor and patient just don't hit it off; there is some undefinable personality clash that prevents a good doctor-patient relationship, and at that juncture they should both bid each other adieu!

I have had the opportunity to recommend many patients for second opinions to individual specialists or to nationally known facilities such as the Mayo Clinic, Scripps Clinic, etc., because these centers have a 'National" name and prominence which many individuals rightfully respect. They may have no different recommendations, but if the patient is reassured, then it's worthwhile. If you're not comfortable with your physician or your treatment, it's your right and responsibility to ask for a second opinion!

Chapter 11
CANCER COMMITTEE

This is the first time, and isn't it a pity,
That anything good came out of committee.
It's really amazing that twelve boring dudes,
Could ever come up with such interesting goods.

The reason is simple, if you look at the members
They're doctors and nurses and laymen and vendors.
And everyone offers their equal two cents
And nobody clamors and nobody vents.

It's a fine honed example without much hypocrisy
Of functioning well in a tiny democracy.
So thank you, dear members, for being so mature
(If you believe this malarkey, I'll sell you manure!)

We have alluded several times to this "Committee", and its importance to a Comprehensive Center for Breast Care. At our medical center, there are several cancer committees for the different specialties such as Gynecologic Oncology (female pelvic organ cancer), Urology, General Cancer, and the Breast Cancer Tumor Committees. They each have a scheduled meeting (working tumor board) where the involved members assemble to discuss cases on a frequent basis. The breast cancer tumor board meets weekly and is represented by many individuals.

The committees may vary, but I will present the members of our committee as an example.

There are one or more of the following: Surgeons (specializing in breast diseases), Medical Oncologists, Family Practice Physicians and General Practitioners, Genetics Oncologists, Radiologists, Radiation Therapists, Pathologists, Plastic Surgeons, Pain Management Specialists (usually Anesthesiologists), Clinical Social Workers,

Oncology Nurses, Tumor Registrars, a Representative from the American Cancer Society, any interested Physicians and Nurses, and a Recording Secretary.

Perhaps the most interesting way to let you know what this committee does is to give you an example of a tumor board case presentation, in brief. If some of the terms sound bizarre, they're probably in the Glossary of Terms. But I just want you to see what we do behind closed doors. For patient privacy, we don't allow the public to be present, and we don't allow the patient to be present so that we can have a free flow of ideas and comments as to treatment and prognosis unhindered by sensitivity to a patient being present.

So, let's begin.

Dr. A (Chairman): "Our first case, Mrs. PDQ is a 56-year-old Caucasian woman who had a screening mammogram on--. Her mother had breast cancer at age 57, had a mastectomy, and is still alive. No other family history of cancer. The patient has been in excellent health with no surgery or medical problems. She had no breast problems; no mass, nipple discharge, skin changes or pain. She is now post menopausal six years, began menses at age twelve, is married and has three children. The rest of the history is negative."

"Can we see the mammograms?"

Dr. B (Radiologist): He places the x-rays on a view box. "As you can see, the left breast is normal. The right breast has several microcalcifications in the upper outer quadrant associated with an area of increased density, measuring about 0.6 centimeters. This area is highly suspicious for malignancy, and a core biopsy was recommended." He takes that x-ray down and places another one. "After discussion with the surgeon and the patient, a stereotactic core biopsy was performed on--with removal of all the microcalcifications in the specimen, and most of the mass effect is now gone. We have placed a metallic clip in the area of the biopsy to mark the location of the original calcifications in case a surgeon has to do a wide excision of the area."

Dr. C (Pathologist): "We received ten small specimens from the core biopsy." She places a slide under the microscope, and this is projected up onto a screen everyone can see. She describes the findings. "We see several areas of atypical ductal hyperplasia, and here is a small focus of invasive ductal carcinoma (cancer) on one of the biopsies. It appears low grade and well differentiated."

Dr. A: "After this report, we discussed the case with the patient and determined she needed a Lumpectomy, sentinel node mapping and sentinel node biopsy, and if the sentinel node was positive, would do an axillary node dissection. The blue dye and radioisotope methods were used, and a solitary sentinel node was isolated, and sent to pathology. A generous lumpectomy was performed. The sentinel node was found to contain a focus of metastatic carcinoma, so a formal axillary dissection was performed. The pathologist will show the slides."

Dr. C: "This is the sentinel node, and as you can see, it shows the small area of metastatic cancer at the rim. We then received the lumpectomy specimen which measured 7 x 6 x 5 centimeters and had a small tumor when it was cut into. The tumor was 1.1 centimeter in diameter, and there was no evidence of other tumor or invasion of the blood vessels. The margins are all free, the narrowest being 1.2 centimeters. We also received a specimen labeled axillary fat pad which contained 18 lymph nodes, all of which were negative." She goes on to describe the microscopic findings, and tells about the various receptors such as estrogen and progesterone being positive.

Dr. A: "Are there any comments from the surgeons? Is any more surgery needed?" They respond that no further surgery is needed since there are adequate, clean margins. "Does this patient need radiation therapy?"

Dr. E (Radiation Therapist): "She will need the standard dose of--rads to the breast after the lumpectomy since the local recurrence rate is about 25% without it. I will not radiate the axilla. The treatment should take about eight weeks, and could be done in conjunction with any chemotherapy."

GP: "When would you start the radiation therapy?"

Dr. E: "When the incisions have healed well--probably about three to four weeks."

Dr. A: "Would the oncologists like to treat this woman?"

Drs. F, G, and H agree: "With a 1.1 centimeter tumor and one positive lymph node, she will need chemotherapy, and since she is ER/PR positive (estrogen and progesterone receptor positive), she should be placed on tamoxifen for five years." They go on to discuss the types of chemotherapy and the dosages.

Dr. A: "Should the radiation and chemotherapy be given at the same time?"

Drs. F, G and H: "Yes. There is no problem with this, and we can start after the wounds heal in about three weeks."

Dr. P (Pain Management Anesthesiologist): "I don't expect this patient to have any significant pain problems that can't be well handled with oral medications such as Vicodin or Darvocet."

Dr. A: "Thank you. What about comments from Psychosocial?"

Ms. L: "I spoke with her and her husband prior to and after the surgery. They seem to be handling the situation well. She has started a lymphedema prevention program with physical therapy, and has been contacted by a representative from Reach To Recovery. She has already attended one of the group discussion meetings and interacts well with the other patients. So far she is doing very well."

Mrs. O (American Cancer Society representative): "She will be introduced to the Wig Bank facilities, and our Look Good Feel Better program in the next few weeks."

Nurse A: "We'll give her a walk-through at the Infusion Center prior to her receiving chemotherapy, and we'll discuss our program with her."

Dr. A: "If there is no further discussion, we will notify her family doctor, the referring surgeon, and her oncologist of our recommendations. Thank you."

And so it is. Of course, this is a very abbreviated version of what occurs, and it's often not so straightforward. Many other issues may be presented and more discussion ensue. But you can get the idea, treatment by discussion with the entire team.

The other benefits are for the group members. I must emphasize that with each case, there is a discussion of the radiology, pathology, and treatment on a more sophisticated level, and it becomes a teaching and learning experience for those present. Better education for the doctors, nurses and other staff means better care for you, the patient It's not uncommon for the general community of physicians to drift away from academics after leaving their training programs, and the Tumor Board offers continuing updates in diagnosis and treatment for all these physicians, and frequently instructs them in areas with which they are not well acquainted.

So, Tumor Boards and Committees benefit the patient and the physicians, nurses, and other staff that are involved in the Comprehensive Breast Center.

(See illustration, next page).

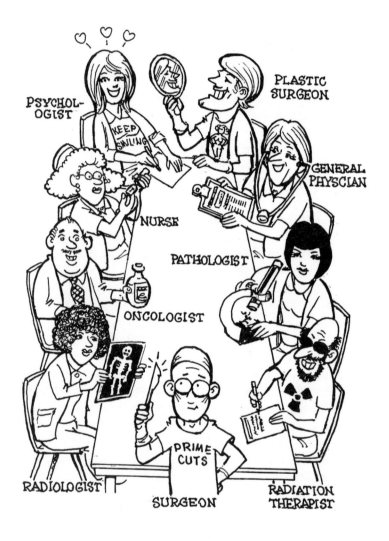

Figure 33. THE CANCER COMMITTEE.

Chapter 12
COMPLEMENTARY
AND ALTERNATIVE METHODS
OF TREATMENT OF BREAST CANCER

Where there is no treatment
There are Many Treatments!

Do you have cancer, come to my store,
I'll sell you some nostrums and tell you some more
Of the grab-bag of treatments you'll find on the shelf
Some sound so good, I take them myself.

These treatments are only for rich educated
They're costly, but cure-alls and NEVER outdated
And since you have cancer your doctor can't cure
Come into my store and I'll fix you for sure.

You say "I'm no fool, I won't fall for this ploy"
Yet it's iron to a magnet or a child to a toy.
Don't underestimate how foolish we'll be
When faced with our imminent mortality.

Well, what's all this stuff about alternative or complementary breast cancer treatments? Let me say at the outset that there are many acceptable, and many unproven and thereby unacceptable treatments that we will be discussing. As I mentioned in the preface, I came to a better understanding of these issues when confronted by a patient seeking out alternative treatment at a Tijuana clinic, and I have prided myself in becoming somewhat of an expert in this field. But knowing the human propensity towards something different and unusual in the face of a challenge, I can understand the popularity of some of the controversial treatments. And whether or not you decide upon these, at least you should be well aware of the pros and cons of the treatments, and know which ones have validity and which ones (in my humble opinion) have none.

I gave a talk on controversial treatment for breast cancer in 1999, and started with the presentation of the word CONVENTIONAL for the therapy offered by differing groups. The most common was the conventional treatments which have come to us through the expertise of the medical CONVENTION of the day, the medicine of physicians and research and the National Cancer Institute supported regimens. The next breakdown was that of the CONVENT or the spiritual and paramedical philosophies--many of which have a great deal of validity as we will see. But this all encompassing word CONVEN-TIONAL also includes another small part which I label the CON part, the side of treatment focusing on unproven, ineffective treatments which bilk the cancer sufferers out of billions of dollars each year, and to which all too many have fallen prey. We have to be careful in not accepting INEXPERT EXPERT ADVICE; it often sounds good, usually too good. And as H.L. Mencken, the writer stated that "For every complex problem there is a simple solution...And it is wrong."

Now let us divide into two areas and define our terms. "Alternative Therapy" is treatment which is prescribed instead of Western Medicine. They are treatments which are unproven because they have not been scientifically tested, or tested and found to be ineffective. They are frequently promoted as cancer cures by people outside the medical profession, and patients suffer either as a direct result of the treatment or because they are doing without legitimate therapy. "Complementary Therapy" is treatment which is, in addition to Western Medicine, using supportive methods which do not cure disease but which control some of the symptoms and improve well-being, and even the length of survival. As you will see, Alternative Therapy often comes under critical scrutiny for its lack of basic research and published support, whereas the latter, while perhaps often not proved in the scientific method, nevertheless works in conjunction with the medically approved standards, and can thereby be of great supplementary help in dealing with the patient with cancer.

"Holistic" medicine is one of these areas which when used as a complementary medical approach can be a significant contribution. These are treatments based on the connection between mind and body and include the following:

Meditation	Music Therapy
Self Help Groups	Acupuncture
Chiropractic	Biofeedback
Yoga	Massage
Stress Management	Homeopathy
Certain Types of Herbal Treatment	

As we will see in the chapter on Psychosocial support groups, we have evidence that those who attend these groups have an increased survival and quality of life, tremendous emotional support, and because of patient-to-patient interaction, often have medical and experiential support which is much needed.

And throughout the United States, there are several Complementary Medicine Programs, among the most noted being at Stanford University with a strong psychosocial program, University of Maryland with stress on mindfulness meditation, relaxation response, and homeopathy, and the Columbia University program which is primarily informational in all aspects of this therapy. Complementary/Alternative Medicine programs (CAM) are taught at the University of Massachusetts by Dr. Jon Kabat-Zinn, at Harvard University by Dr. Herbenson, and at the University of Arizona by Dr. Andrew Weil. Other university programs offer multiple therapies including Massage, Herbs, Qigong (a good Scrabble word!), chiropractic, mindfulness, and T'ai Chi.

Linda Pearson, Editor-in-Chief of *The Nurse Practitioner*, gave a very insightful look at alternative medicine with her statement that, "Some of the movement toward 'alternative' medicine reflects a current trend in society toward rejecting 'science' as a method of ascertaining truths."*

* Editor's Memo, *Nurse Practitioner*, November, 1998, article: Alternative Therapy: Cautionary Tale, Linda Pearson, RN, SNP, MSN, Editor-in-Chief of *Nurse Practitioner*.

Let us look into some of these CAM therapies, and hopefully dissect the valued from the valueless. Of course, I cannot give detailed analyses of all these treatments in this review, but suffice it so say, the Information Centers can find data for and against these treatments if sought.

We will look at Diet and Nutrition therapies such as the macrobiotic diet, the Gerson diet, and others including vitamins and minerals. There are the Mind-Body techniques such as biofeedback, relaxation and guided imagery, meditation, hypnosis, yoga, and support groups which we know to be very beneficial. Then Bioelectromagnetics including acupuncture, homeopathy, and "laying of hands", and the Traditional medicines from other cultures such as Indian Ayurvedic medicine, Chinese and other Asian medicines. We will take a close look at the very questionable Pharmacological and Biological therapies including Shark Cartilage, Laetrile, and Krebiozen. Then there is the Manual Healing with well respected physical therapy, massage, therapeutic touch, and chiropractic techniques, And finally, herbal medicine such as that practiced by native American Shamans and indigenous healers.

But first let us look at the individuals who are utilizing the most extreme of the alternative therapies. It's interesting to know that the largest percentage of users are from the group with a household income greater than $50,000, and that more users come from those with a higher level of education, i.e., 5% did not complete high school whereas 13% had completed graduate or professional school. And we are flooded with an overabundance of nonscientific rationales for undertaking these programs:

> *"My aunt and several of her friends have been treated and cured by this."*
> *"Don't rely just on science--look into yourselves for the cure--your body can cure itself."*
> *"Your mother should have come to us sooner. Your regular doctors have destroyed her normal immune system. But we may still be able to help."*
> *" My oncologist says I am incurable but my healer says that this is not so; therefore I'm not going back to my oncologist."*

"Physicians only have expensive treatments, whereas alternative treatments are relatively cheap."
"All doctors want to do is make money at my expense."

Now let us examine some of the more popular treatments.

The Rife Research Laboratory indicates that it has one of the greatest health discoveries in history, and that it has been suppressed by the medical community. They claim that a revolutionary microscope discovered in the 1920's by Royal Raymond Rife, Jr., may be a cure for all types of infectious diseases, and that by using radio frequencies, they can actually arrest most cancers and even cure them. They even use a quote from Victor Hugo to support their theories: "An idea whose time has come is stronger than armies!" And after stating how valuable their treatment was, they are quick to state that, "Due to FDA regulations and various state laws, no medical claims can be made for the use of magnetic polarizers, and that these magnets must be for experimental research only!" However, their brochure follows with several pages of the appropriate programs and frequencies for treating and possibly curing such diverse problems as General Cancer and Breast Cancer, Boils, AIDS, Obesity, Rheumatism, Hair Loss, Malaria, Tuberculosis, Shingles, and Yellow Fever. The brochure is complete with attestations by cured patients, and the PFG-100 Frequency Instrument (plus user's guide) is available for $2,495 along with magnetic polarizers for $130 each.

For many of the alternative treatments, I will give comments on their validity but I won't even attempt to justify any comments about the Rife magnetic polarizer. I leave it to you to make your own evaluation if you like.

We can even find the extremes of treatment philosophy in the little booklet by Anonymous Star entitled, "Cancer Is Good For You", in which the author questions our entire scientific basis of cancer by stating that cancer is the result of what he describes as organo-muta-genesis or a body's attempt to correct abnormal chemistry (the result of unhealthful habits) by generating a New Organ to correct the abnormal blood chemistry. The pamphlet ends with a song entitled "Cancer is Good For You". I am not even arguing the validity of such publications except to say that before one undertakes to accept a new or questionable treatment, do yourself a big favor, and look into the data that will support such treatment. Yes, some of the spiritual and psychosocial supports advocated are certainly beneficial (*see* the chapter on Psychosocial Support) but care must be taken to move more towards the conventional than the "convent" or the "con" if we are truly seeking good medical help.

The Mexican Border Clinics have been studied by the National Cancer Institute, and they have found no objective evidence to support various procedures known as "metabolic therapies" advocated by many of these groups. Metabolic therapy has three phases, according to its proponents; Detoxification, including fasting and bowel cleansing; Strengthening the immune system with numerous supplements; and Attacking Cancer with natural and nontoxic chemicals. They advocate the use of Hydrogen peroxide, pressed liver, carrot juice, coffee enemas, Laetrile, massive doses of vitamins, and other pseudoscientific regimes. Many individuals are told they have pre-cancer and are given regimens to prevent cancer; others are misdiagnosed as having cancer and having remarkable cures. A great deal of evaluation has been done on most of these treatments, and none of them has been found to be of any significant value in controlled clinical trials. Some are even dangerous!

The appeal of these clinics is that they offer a loving, warm, and tender environment, and an approach to treatment (at high cost) offering cures to desperate individuals who will overlook reality in an attempt to prolong their lives. The National Cancer Institute and the American Cancer Society have voluminous amounts of information debunking much of the treatment advocated.

And treatment is not cheap, averaging from $2500 to $4500 per day. Although the clinics state that they are paid in cash "up front", they insist that most of the treatment is covered by insurance. Patients find out too late that the cost, in most instances, is not reimbursable, and I have known individuals who have mortgaged their homes and used up their savings for a last chance at a cure.

Now let us look at some of the specific drugs.

Laetrile, called "vitamin B17", has been extensively tested by reputable organizations including the National Cancer Institute (NCI), and found to be totally ineffective as a treatment for cancer (researchers have even found high levels of cyanide in the blood of many patients treated with this drug!). NCI-sponsored clinical trials of "anti-neoplastins" promoted by Dr. Stanislaw Burzynski of the Burzynski Research Institute, and Dr. Harold Manner's metabolic program for the treatment of cancer (enzyme and vitamin therapy, fasting and coffee enemas) have found no scientific basis for these treatments, and no effective way of treating cancer. Yet the educated public still line up to get the treatment as a last resort or in many cases, as a first and only resort, often losing the opportunity for treatment and cure by conventional methods.

Dr. Koch's Synthetic antitoxins (Malonide, Glyoxylide, and Parabenzoquinone) supposedly stimulate the destruction of cancer--causing toxins. Frequently, the exact contents of the treatments is kept secret to prevent "sabotage" by the medical establishment.

Krebiozen, originally an extract from horse serum devised by Dr. Steven Durovic and Dr. Andrew Ivy, has undergone extensive testing, and found to have no proven anticancer activity. Similarly, the Gerson Diet stressed that a natural diet would counteract years of bad nutrition in curing cancer, and advocated fresh calve's liver juice, vitamins, minerals, and thyroid extract and coffee enemas. Salt and spices, and even aluminum utensils could not be used. No proved efficacy of this diet has been shown. Dr. Lawrence Burton established The Immunology Researching Center in the Bahamas in 1977 with a treatment called Immunoaugmentative Therapy (IAT) which he claimed was effective against cancer, multiple sclerosis, and acquired immunodeficiency syndrome (AIDS). Although he has described success in treating cancer patients in the media, he has never subjected his work to critical scientific evaluation, and so IAT must be considered as unproved and of questionable value.

Virginia Livingston-Wheeler of the Livingston-Wheeler Clinic believed that cancer is caused by a bacterium, "Progenitor cryptocides", when the body's normal immune system was flawed. Her treatment, involving vaccines, antibiotics, and enzymes, and a low-carbohydrate diet, has no scientific support from the NCI or other sources. Likewise, a substance called Cancell or Entelev developed by Mr. James V. Sheridan, a mixture of chemicals combined on the basis of some electrical activity, could cure cancer as well as AIDS, Epstein-Barr virus and Herpes virus. There is no scientific support for this treatment either.

The whole area of Holistic Medicine includes a wide variety of philosophies and practices, and the basic principle of considering each patient as a functioning whole, spiritual, mental, physical, and emotional has shown to be of importance from a psychosocial point of view. As is shown in our "Psychosocial" chapter, these approaches must be evaluated on an individual basis, and used in conjunction with accepted medical care to be of true value to the patient with cancer. The NCI finds the following Nutritional Therapies of questionable value, and they should be carefully examined with your own physician before undertaken. These include Vitamin C, Hoxsey Herbal, Gerson Diet, Manner Metabolic Diet, Pao D'Arco Tea, Macro-Biotic Diets, Kelley Metabolic Diet, and Ozone Treatments.

So what should the inquiring patient do to evaluate the validity of treatments? It is important to base the decision on a rational approach, proven, clinically-tested studies, and what we consider clinical trial validated methods. No sensible person can really believe that there is a hidden agenda by the medical profession to cover up a cure for cancer so that doctors can line their purses. Perhaps just the opposite holds true. Charlatans and the worse type of "mountebanks" approach the cancer patient at his or her most vulnerable stage through print or word of mouth, or through the voices of those who have been "taken in" by the claims, to extract money from the unsuspecting individuals. It is a sad but true reflection on the society of today.

We should ask the following questions about any treatment being offered, both conventional and non-conventional.

Is the treatment available for public scrutiny, and has it undergone clinical trials by major medical centers and reputable researchers?

Is it a treatment solely based on diet therapy, excluding standard medical regimens? (There is no evidence to show that diet alone can cure cancer!)

Is the treatment offered with concomitant accusations against the standard medical community, downplaying or negating years of valid clinical scientific trials?

Does the treatment claim to be inexpensive, harmless, painless, secretive or so bizarre as to raise a red flag? (Cancer treatment is a difficult undertaking because, in effect, the treatments given are destroying cancerous tissue in the body, and this involves powerful medicines with frequent negative side effects.) The easier, softer way, while more appealing, may have no value whatsoever.

So let me conclude by saying that it is the responsibility of the patient and the patient's family as well as the patient's physician to steer her or him toward a valid program of treatment which includes a solidly-based medical treatment, and a strong psychosocial program to effect the best possible outcome with the least morbidity and suffering. The information available through an Information Center such as those in the American Cancer Society offices can be examined through literature and computer data. Don't take my word for it. If presented with alternative treatments, use the resources available to find out about them, and be able to make an informed and intelligent decision.

Dr. Michael Baum, ChM, FRCS, has graciously allowed me to use a "Table of A to Z of unproven methods of cancer diagnosis and treatment" from his article of "Quack cancer cures or scientific remedies".* It seems an appropriate way to finish this article.

TABLE of A to Z of unproven methods of cancer diagnosis and treatment.

A Aromatherapy, acupuncture
B Bach's flower remedy

C Christian science, chiro-
crystal healing, carrot juice

D Dousing
E Vitamin E, electroacupuncture
F Faith healing, fire walking
G Gerson therapy
H Homeopathy, herbalism
I Iscador, iridology
J Johnson's remedy
K Krebiozen
L Laetrile
M Moxibustion

N Negative ionizers
O Osteopathy, organic diet orgone
accumulators

P Psychic surgery, psionic medicine
medicine, pyramidology Pauling's
vitamin C cure

Q Quinine
R Radionics, reflexology
S Simonton's cure, selenium
T Theosophy, tai chi, trepanation
U Urine therapy
V Vrilium tubes, vegatest
W Water remedy
X Xanthine remedy
Y Yoga
Z Zinc, zebethium occidentale

• With permission from Michael Baum, ChM, FRCS, *Journal of the Royal Society of Medicine*, October, 1996, article: "Quack cancer cures or scientific remedies".

Chapter 13
PATHOLOGY

In 1674, Leeuwenhoek conjured up the microscope
And saw a lot of tiny germs and wonders of a cornucope,
It's all been history since then, you'll see,
He started the field of pathology.

A strange group of doctors who hid in dark rooms
Avoiding the sunlight and grave-robbing tombs,
They derived satisfaction from seeing dead bodies
And looked in their 'scopes while they downed their hot-toddies.

And now they make slides out of tissue and bugs
That they find in your body or under your rugs,
They're able with skill to tell with a smile
Whether you're human or just a reptile.

You may ask: "So what? I don't care what they find."
That just shows that you have a very small mind
Cause these are the people with lenses and knife
Who help us to look at the basis of life.

They can tell in a moment benign from malignant
(Don't question them or they'll become quite indignant.)
And depending upon whether they give the right answer
Is whether or not you are treated for cancer!

This is the section of the book which may seem cloaked in mystery. Pathology is the branch of medicine that deals with abnormality or variation from the normal. If normal puts one at ease-then this is dis-ease. The pathologists are physicians who must completely understand the normal to be able to differentiate it from the abnormal and they are in many ways the "toti-potential" physicians with their "fingers in every pot". And remember, they not only do tissue examination with slides under the microscope, they are also in charge of the clinical laboratory that evaluates blood and urine and other body samples and run all the esoteric studies that let your doctor know what's going on in your body. Each doctor, whether primary care or specialist, depends on the expertise of the pathologist to guide them in their treatment.

The pathologists are the unseen physicians in most institutions and most patients never see or speak with them. Fortunately, at some centers such as our own, some of the pathologists make themselves available to patients to discuss their pathology and sometimes even show them tissue specimens and microscopic tissues which are not only interesting, but give the patient a better understanding of her own disease whether it be benign or malignant. Such an individual is pathologist, Dr. Kamini Malhotra, who has an open door policy to physicians and patients alike. She also speaks to the Breast Cancer Support groups and brings into the light of day a field heretofore mysterious and foreign to the general public. It is a privilege to present her section on Pathology of Breast Cancer.

Now, to many of you this chapter may seem very complex. I have to emphasize that this is one area where it is important to be very complete. You may want to read it all at once or you may just read certain sections which pertain to your particular interest.

PATHOLOGY OF BREAST CANCER

Breast cancer is the most common type of cancer among women in the U.S., other than skin cancer. Knowledge about breast cancer is increasing. Cancer research has led to real progress against breast cancer. There is better survival and improved quality of life. Breast Cancer also occurs in males. Much of the information on the symptoms, diagnosis and treatment, and living with breast cancer applies to men as well as women.

What is cancer?
Cancer is a group of different diseases that have some important things in common. They arise in cells--the bodies' basic unit of life. The body is made up of many types of cells. To understand different types of cancer, it is helpful to know about normal cells and what

happens when they become cancerous. Normally cells grow and divide to produce more cells only when the body needs them. This orderly process helps keep the body healthy. Sometimes the cells keep dividing when new cells are not needed and these cells can form a mass of tissue growth, which is new and can be called the *neoplasm* or *tumor.* Neoplasm literally means "new growth" and represents uncoordinated tissue growth that persists in an excessive manner, after cessation of stimuli, which evokes the change.

This abnormal mass is purposeless and preys on the host and is virtually autonomous. Tumors can be benign or malignant. In the majority of cases one can differentiate a benign tumor from a malignant tumor with considerable certainty.

The characteristics of benign tumors and malignant tumors are based on differentiation of the cell, that is, the extent to which the neoplastic cells resemble comparable normal cells.

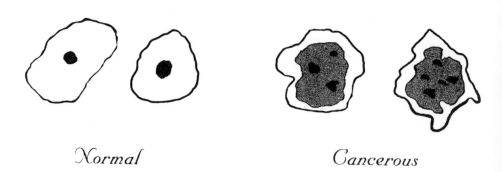

$\mathcal{N}ormal$ $\mathcal{C}ancerous$

Figure 34. NORMAL AND ABNORMAL CELLS.

Benign tumors grow very slowly over a period of years, whereas cancers grow rapidly. Benign tumors do not invade other tissue structures and will generally be encapsulated.

Malignant tumors show less differentiation. They grow rapidly, spread to other parts of the body and form secondary tumors, which are called Metastases.

Pathways of spread:
Dissemination of cancer occurs through:
1. Direct seeding of body cavities and surfaces.
2. Lymphatic spread (through lymph vessels).
3. Hematogenous spread (through blood vessels).

Carcinogenesis:
Carcinogenesis that is formation of cancer, is a multi-step process. Genetic damages are at the heart of carcinogenesis. The principal targets of genetic damage are two classes of normal regulatory genes, the growth promoting proto-oncogenes and the
growth inhibiting cancer suppressor genes (anti-oncogenes). A third category of genes, those that control programmed cell deaths or apoptosis, are also important in carcinogenesis.

The Natural History:
The natural history of malignant tumors can be divided into four phases.
1. Malignant change (transformation of a normal cell into a malignant cell)
2. Growth of these transformed cells
3. Local invasion
4. Distant metastases

How long does it take to produce a clinically overt tumor mass? It has been calculated that a transformed cell must undergo at least 30 population doublings to produce a mass weighing 1 gram, which is the smallest detectable mass clinically.

Anatomy and Histology of Normal Breast:
The resting mammary gland consists of 6-10 major duct systems, each of which is divided into lobes, and lobules that are the functional units. Thin tubes called ducts link all the lobes and lobules. These ducts lead to the nipple in the center of dark area of skin called the

areola. Fat fits the spaces around the lobules and the ducts. There are no muscles in the breast. The muscles lie underneath each breast and cover the ribs.

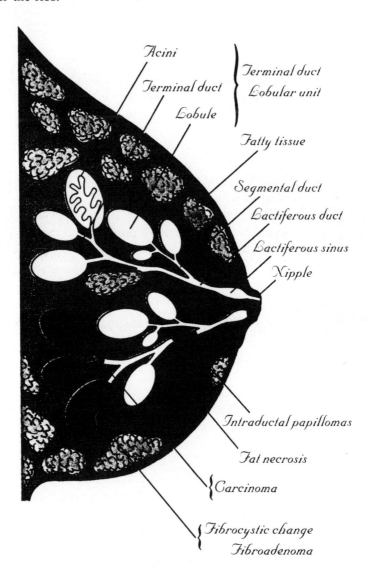

Figure 35. THE ANATOMY OF THE BREAST.

Each breast also carries blood vessels that carry colorless fluid called lymph. The lymph vessels lead to small bean-shaped organs called lymph nodes. Clusters of lymph nodes are found near the breast in the axilla (under the arm), above the collarbone and in the chest. These are regional lymph nodes. Lymph nodes are also found in many other parts of the body.

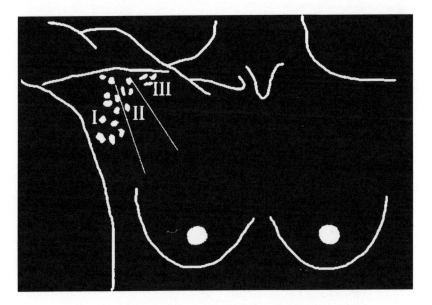

Figure 36. REGIONAL AXILLARY LYMPH NODES, LEVELS 1,2,3.

Before puberty the complex system of branching ducts ends blindly. At menarche it proliferates distally and gives rise to some 30 epithelial-lined ductules. Each terminal duct and ductule compose the terminal ductal lobular unit. Just as the endometrium rises at each menstrual cycle, so does the breast. The stimulatory effect of estrogen and progesterone accounts for the sense of fullness commonly experienced by women during the premenstrual phase of cycle. With onset of pregnancy the breast assumes its complete morphologic maturation and functional activity. Following lactation the gland regresses and atrophies but never back to the virginal state. After the third decade the ducts and lobules further atrophy with shrinkage of the stroma and replacement by fat.

Benign Breast Diseases

The following conditions fall under this category. These are conditions commonly experienced.

1. Acute mastitis or inflammation and breast abscess
2. Fat necrosis
3. Fibrocystic disease

Fibrocystic disease applies to miscellaneous changes in the female breast that range from those that are, entirely innocuous to those that are, associated with increased risk of cancer. There is usually cyst formation with fibrosis and some hyperplasia of the ducts and lobules as well as another condition, of sclerosing adenosis. Together these variants comprise the single most common disorder of the breast and account for more than one-half of all the surgical operations on the female breast. About 10% of the women develop clinically apparent cystic disease. The condition is unusual before adolescence. It is usually seen between the ages of 20 and 40 and peaks at or just before menopause. Hormonal imbalances are considered to be basic, to the development of this disorder. The clinical significance of fibrocystic changes is that they can produce masses in the breast that require differentiation from cancer. It can have microcalcifications within it that are detected on mammography and some of these conditions may predispose to subsequent development of cancer.

Benign Tumors Fibroadenoma:

Fibroadenoma is the most common benign tumor of the female breast. It is a growth composed of fibrous and glandular tissues and presents as a spherical nodule that is usually sharply circumscribed and freely mobile. Slight increases in size may occur during late phases of each menstrual cycle. Pregnancy can stimulate its growth. At menopause regression or calcification can occur.

Phyllodes Tumor:

Phyllodes tumors, like Fibroadenomas, arise from intralobular tissues and, resemble a Fibroadenoma. They can be fairly large in size. They are much less common than a Fibroadenoma. The majority of these tumors are benign, however these tumors may recur or they can be frankly malignant.

Intraductal Papilloma:

Intraductal papilloma is a neoplastic papillary growth within a duct and clinically they can present as bloody discharge from the nipple, or a small subareolar tumor, or as nipple retraction. These benign tumors can be excised to prevent local recurrences.

Risk Factors:

The cancer committee of the College of American Pathologists has prepared an update of the consensus statement on pre-malignant breast lesions and breast cancer risk that was originally published in 1986. The objective of this publication was to better define the relative risk associated with specific histologic conditions.

Relative risk for developing invasive breast cancer is based on pathologic exam of benign breast tissues.

A. *No Increased Risks:*
1. Sclerosing adenosis
2. Duct ectasia
3. Fibroadenoma without complex features
4. Fibrosis
5. Mastitis
6. Mild hyperplasia without atypia
7. Ordinary cysts
8. Apocrine metaplasia
9. Squamous metaplasia

B. *Slightly increased risk* -1.5 to 2.0 times.
1. Fibroadenoma with complex features.
2. Moderate or florid hyperplasia without atypia
3. Sclerosing adenosis when present with atypical ductal hyperplasia
4. Solitary papilloma with co-existent atypical ductal hyperplasia

C. *Moderately increased risk* - 4.0 to 5.0 times.
1. Atypical ductal hyperplasia
2. Atypical lobular hyperplasia

D. *Markedly increased risk* - 8.0 to 10.0 times.
Ductal carcinoma in situ
Lobular carcinoma in situ

Specific probability of developing breast cancer in the next 10 years.

Current age in years	No increased risk	2x increased risk	4x increased risk
20	1/2000	1/1000	1/500
30	1/256	1/128	1/64
40	1/67	1/34	1/17
50	1/39	1/20	1/110
60	1/29	1/15	1/7

Breast Cancer:

Breast cancer causes about 16% of cancer deaths among females and has been called the foremost cancer in women. The incidence has been increasing steadily over the past 80 years such that currently one out of every 8 women in the United States will develop cancer in their lifetime. Understandably, breast cancer has received a great deal of appropriate publicity and has been the focus of intensive study. Although much is gained particularly in early diagnosis, the age-adjusted death rate from breast cancer has virtually remained the same over the past 30 years. This year, in 1999, 176,300 new cases are expected out of which 1300 are male breast cancers. The estimated number of cancer deaths in 1999 due to breast cancer is 43,700 out of which 400 are male breast cancers. Breast Cancer is the second most common cause of cancer deaths in women, Lung cancer being number one. It is ironic that a tumor arising in an exposed organ readily accessible to self-examination and clinical diagnosis continues to exact such a heavy toll.

At the time of diagnoses:
• 65% of breast cancer is localized, that is confined to the breast.
• 29% of the time it shows spread to the regional lymph nodes.
• 6% of the time it shows evidence of distant spread.
Five-year survival rate for all stages of breast cancer is about 87%.
  • 98% for localized disease
  • 78% for regional disease
  • 28% for distant disease

Incidence and Epidemiology

Cancer of the female breast is rarely found before the age of 25 except in certain familial cases. It can occur at any age thereafter with a peak incidence at or after menopause. It is 5 times more common in the United States than in Japan and Taiwan.

1. *Genetic pre-disposition is well defined.*
   85% of breast cancers are sporadic. 10-15% are hereditary. The magnitude of risk is in proportion to the number of close relatives with breast cancer and the age when cancer occurred in the relative. The younger the relative at the time of development of cancer, the greater the genetic predisposition. The risk is 1.5 to 2.0 x more for women with a first degree relative with breast cancer, and 4-6 times more for those with 2 affected relatives. There are uncommon high-risk families with apparent autosomal dominant transmission and familial association of breast and ovarian carcinomas. Breast cancer affects 25% of patients with the Li/Fraumeni syndrome (multiple sarcomas and carcinomas) and is associated with germ line mutations of tumor suppressor gene P53. Breast Cancer genes implicated are:

   BRCA1 gene   Onchromosome 17q 21 associated with ovarian cancer

   BRCA2 gene   Onchromosome 13q 12/13

2. *Increasing age.*
   It is uncommon before the age of 25. There is a steady rise to the time of menopause followed by a slower rise throughout life.

3. *Length of reproductive life.*
   The risk increases with early menarche and late menopause.

4. *Parity.*
   It is more frequent in nulliparous women than in multiparous women.

5. *Age at first childbirth.*
   There is increased risk when older than 30 years of age at the time of first child.

6. *Obesity.*
   Increased risk is attributed to synthesis of estrogens and fat depots.

7. *Exogenous estrogens.*

There is moderately increased risk with hormone therapy for menopausal symptoms.

8. *Oral contraceptives.*

There is no clear-cut risk attributed to balanced content of estrogens and progesterones currently used in oral contraceptives.

9. *Fibrocystic change with atypical ductal hyperplasia.*

(*see* above chart). Also carries increased risk.

10. *Cancer of the contralateral breast or* endometrium.

Also carries an increased risk.

11. *Radiation therapy.*

Women, whose breasts are exposed to radiation during childhood (especially those who are treated for Hodgkin's lymphoma) are at increased risk for developing breast cancer throughout their lives. Studies show that a younger a woman was when radiation was given, the higher the risk for developing breast cancer.

Etiology and Pathogenesis

The epidemiological data points to three sets of influences that may be important in breast cancer.

1. Genetic factors
2. Hormonal imbalances
3. Environmental factors

The genetic factors and hormonal imbalances have been addressed above.

Environmental influences.

Various items and diets have been implicated, but the role of high fat diet previously well accepted is now questioned. Coffee addicts will be pleased to know that there is no substantial evidence that caffeine consumption increases the risk. Studies suggest that moderate alcohol consumption is associated with a 1.5 increased risk of breast cancer. The virus called Mouse Mammary Tumor Virus (a retrovirus) was implicated in the past, but the findings have not been conclusive.

More is being learned of the possible contributions of oncogenes and tumor suppressor genes to breast cancer in particular. Application of the erb/B2/neu gene which is similar to the gene for the receptor to Epidermal Growth Factor (EGF) is found in from 5% to as many as 30% of the cancers associated with over-expression of the protein seen in carcinoma cells. Over-expression of the gene is associated with poor prognosis in patients with lymph node positive breast cancer. Amplification of the Int/2, C/ras and C/myc has also been implicated. Finally somatic mutations of P53 and Rb suppressor genes occur in 50% and 20% of breast cancers respectively.

Classification and Distribution

Breast cancer is more common in the left breast than the right. 50% of them arise in the upper outer quadrant (UOQ), 10% in upper inner quadrant (UIQ), 10% in lower inner quadrant (LIQ), and 10% in lower outer quadrant (LOQ) and 20% in the central or subareolar region. Tumors are classified in certain categories.

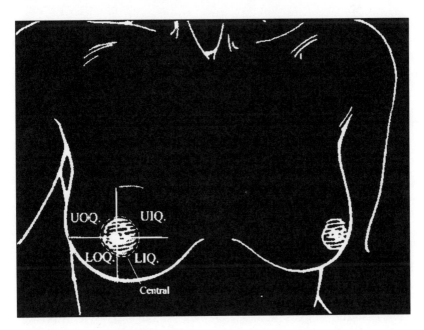

Figure 37. Locations in the Breast. UOQ = Upper outer quadrant. UIQ = Upper inner quadrant. LOQ = Lower outer quadrant. LIQ = Lower inner quadrant.

The World Health Organization classification is as follows:
Non-invasive tumors
  1. Intraductal carcinoma (Ductal carcinoma in situ)
  2. Intraductal carcinoma with Paget's disease

3. Lobular carcinoma in situ

Invasive breast cancer
1. Invasive Ductal carcinoma NOS
2. Invasive Ductal carcinoma with Paget's disease
3. Invasive lobular carcinoma
4. Medullary carcinoma
5. Colloid carcinoma
6. Tubular carcinoma
7. Adenoid cystic carcinoma
8. Apocrine carcinoma
9. Invasive papillary carcinoma

The most common tumor, however, is invasive Ductal carcinoma.

Ductal carcinoma in situ (DCIS)

Ductal carcinoma in situ is a form of malignant transformation of the epithelial cells lining the mammary ducts and lobules. The proliferating cells are confined by an intact basement membrane. That is, there is no demonstrable evidence of break down of the basement membrane and spilling of these cancerous cells into the adjacent tissue (infiltration) by light microscopy.

Although Ductal carcinoma in situ is a precursor of invasive carcinoma, not all patients will progress to invasive cancer. The percentage of Ductal carcinoma in situ that progress to invasion is unknown since the natural history remains unclear. Those who do develop it, will do so in 5-10 years in the same site. Microinvasion is seen in about 1.8% of patients with microcalcifications and about 1% of patients with Ductal carcinoma in situ have spread of tumor into the lymph nodes in the armpit (axillary lymph node metastases) which is an undetected consequence of tissue invasion.

Distribution of Ductal carcinoma in situ is of considerable interest. Several studies suggest that Ductal carcinoma in situ is a multicentric disease, however recent studies, using pathologic mammographic correlative techniques have shown that the additional foci are almost always present in relation to the index lesion (multifocal spread).

Most Ductal carcinoma in situs have a segmental pattern of involvement in the breast. A surgical procedure of segmentectomy would be ideal, though it is difficult to perform a segmentectomy, according to a number of experienced breast surgeons. These observations favor that breast preserving features may be feasible in many patients.

Ductal carcinoma is a heterogeneous disease. Its subtypes differ with respect to histology, mammography, clinical presentation and biologic behavior. The classification is designed to predict the outcome of the disease.

Ductal carcinoma in situ is classified into different subtypes based upon its architectural features.

1. Comedo features with comedo type. This accounts for 40-50% of the cases.
2. Non-comedo type under which fall the following categories:
   - Cribriform types solid type and micropapillary type

A grading scheme must recognize subtypes with significant differences in outcome. It must be simple to use, and must be reproducible in clinical practice. Grading of Ductal carcinoma in situ has become a part of standard practice in clinical management of Ductal carcinoma in situ and should be done routinely. Three nuclear grades are described--Nuclear grade 1, Grade 2, and Grade 3. Necrosis is considered present for any architectural pattern of Ductal carcinoma in situ in which central lumina contain necrotic neoplastic cells.

Pathologic classification score Pathologic Classification score is obtained by using two features.

1. Nuclear grade.
2. Comedo type necrosis.

Features of Ductal carcinoma in situ, comedo type are frequently associated with a high nuclear grade, aneuploidy, high proliferation rate, HER-2/neu (see erb/2 gene amplification or protein over-expression and more aggressive clinical behavior). Non-comedo type of Ductal carcinoma in situ is just the opposite.

In the past, mastectomy was the gold standard for Ductal carcinoma in situ, "doing more surgery for less disease" and thus effecting a 98%-to 100% cure rate but as less and less is being done for invasive breast cancer, the treatment for Ductal carcinoma in situ is also turning do doing less. Lumpectomies are considered more and more for this condition.

Van Nuys prognostic index (VNPI) was developed to aid in the complex treatment selection process for Ductal carcinoma in situ and is only a guideline. In this scheme, points are scored based on 3 predictors of local recurrence.
1. Pathologic grade of tumor.
2. Size of tumor.
3. Surgical margins around tumor.
Scores of 1 (are the best) to 3 (being the worst) are assigned for each of the 3 predictors and then totaled to give an overall VNPI score ranging from 3 to 9.

The final formula for the VNPI **equals pathologic classification score, plus margin score plus size score.** The VNPI guideline can be used to help selection of treatment. For example DCIS patients with VNPI scores of 3 or 4 may be treated with excision alone. DCIS patients with VNPI scores of 5, 6, or 7 may be treated with excision and radiation, and DCIS patients with VNPI scores of 8 or 9 should be considered for mastectomy. With a diagnosis of ductal carcinoma in situ, the pathology report should contain the following information:

1. The site and quadrant
2. Pathologic subtype and nuclear grade
3. Presence of comedo necrosis
4. Size and extent of lesion
5. Margins
6. Degree of association between Ductal carcinoma in situ and mammographic microcalcification.
7. Include reason for and type of biopsy, for example, palpable abnormality of mammographic microcalcification.
8. Stereotactic core biopsy versus excisional biopsy.

Certain prognostic factors are important in predicting recurrence of Ductal carcinoma in situ.
1. Tumor size/margin with nuclear grade
2. Van Nuys classification
3. Comedo necrosis
4. Architecture
5. Residual Ductal carcinoma in situ at excision
6. Lymphocytic infiltration, fibrosis

7. Suspicious mammograms
8. Microcalcification
9. Age
10. Pathologically palpable versus non-palpable

Lobular carcinoma in situ (LCIS)

Lobular carcinoma in situ is a histologically unique lesion manifested by a proliferation in one or more terminal ducts and/or ductules. These lesions can be seen in breasts removed for fibrocystic disease in the vicinity of invasive carcinoma, with sclerosing adenosis and fibroadenoma. In patients not treated with mastectomy and followed for 24 years, the frequency of second carcinoma developing in the same or contralateral breast was 30%. The risk is eight to ten times greater than that expected for the general population. Infiltrating carcinoma that develops is either ductal or lobular. The lesion is thus a marker for invasive carcinoma. The risk of developing invasive Ductal carcinoma is one percent per year or ten percent per ten year.

Invasive Breast Cancer

Invasive Ductal carcinomas account for 65% to 80% of all mammary cancers. These growths occur as sharply limited nodules of stony-hard consistency that average 1- 2 cm. in size and rarely exceed 4-5 cm. On palpation they may have an infiltrative attachment to the surrounding structures with fixation to the underlying chest wall, dimpling of the skin, and retraction of the nipple. The mass is characteristic on cut section, is retracted below the cut surface and has a hard consistency and produces a grating sound when cut.

Breast Cancer is a heterogeneous and progressive disease and requires multidisciplinary diagnosis and treatment. There are many types of breast cancer that have different growth rates, malignancy grades and mammographic/clinical appearances and outcomes. The possibility of controlling breast cancer through detection and treatment at its early stages can be considered one of the most important achievements in cancer research over the past 3 decades.

With early diagnosis, when size of tumor is small, and with early treatment, the natural history of the disease can be altered. Therefore, emphasis should be placed on detecting the disease years before it becomes palpable. Screening with mammography during the past 30 years has shown a significant decrease in mortality from breast cancer. The beneficial effect of screening is mediated via its effect on tumor size, histologic grade and node status. Tumor size increases with time. Node status (that is, involvement of the lymph nodes) is also a time-related tumor characteristic.

Prognosis

Once the diagnosis is made, either on a stereotactic core needle biopsy or excisional biopsy of the lump, the treatment decisions are based on several prognostic factors:

Size of primary tumor - The diameter of the tumor shows a good correlation with the presence or absence of spread to regional lymph nodes (nodal spread) and the survival rate. The smaller the size of the tumor at the time of diagnosis the lower the grade of the tumor and therefore less chance of spread to the regional lymph nodes. Tumors under one centimeter in size or less with negative regional lymph nodes have an excellent survival: 92% at ten years.

1. Lymph node involvement - (Negative nodes 80% 5 year survival, 1-3 positive nodes 50% survival). Lymph node involvement has a profound influence on survival. The axillary lymph node status is the single most important prognostic factor for patients with early breast cancer. There is a sharp difference in survival rates between patients with positive and negative nodes. Survival rate also depends in the level of axillary lymph nodes involved as well, that is either level 1, 2, or 3, Level 1 being nearest to the breast tissue and Level 3 being the furthest away from the breast tissue. The number of lymph nodes involved is also important: less than 4 or greater than 4. For prognostic purposes, the best grouping is as follows:

• Negative nodes
• 1-3 nodes positive
• or more nodes positive

Patients who have lymph nodes that are negative on light microscopy but are found to have micrometastases later by special studies have the same prognosis as patients in whom no tumor is found in the lymph nodes. Even so, 20-30% of patients with negative nodes suffer recurrence and die of their disease in 10 years. Because of this, there is a continuing search for better biological markers of diagnosis. In summary, small tumors with negative nodes have:

Stage 1.
• a 10 year disease-free survival of 92%
• a 20 year disease-free survival of 88%

Stage IIA and I (lymph node involvement have)
• a 10 year disease-free interval of 71%
• a 20 year disease-free interval of 66%
• 2-4 lymph node involved
• 10 and 20 year survival of 62% and 56%
  More than 4 lymph nodes involved
• 10 and 20-year disease free rates are 47% and 43%

2. Histologic grade and type of tumor - Microscopic grade. The most widely used microscopic grading system is that of Bloom and Richardson and is based on the architectural pattern of the tumor, on the degree of nuclear atypia and the number of mitotic figures seen per 10hpf. The utility of this system has been repeatedly proved.

3. Margins - Tumors with pushing margins have a better prognosis than tumors with infiltrating margins.

4. Necrosis - The presence of necrosis is associated with increased incidence of lymph node involvement and decreased survival.

5. Presence/absence of estrogen receptors and progesterone receptors - Patients with estrogen receptor positive tumors determined by immunohistochemistry have a longer disease-free survival than others.

6. Proliferative rate of tumors and aneuploidy - DNA ploidy. It is not yet clear whether this parameter adds independent information of prognostic value once the size of the tumor, the grade of the tumor, lymph node status and hormone receptor status are taken into account.

7. Presence of amplified or activated oncogenes C/erb 2(neu/-HER/oncogene) - Amplification of this oncogene is seen in almost all cases of comedo-type intraductal carcinoma and in 30% of invasive ductal cases, and in very rare cases of invasive lobular cancers. This is also detected by immunohistochemical studies. The amplification of this oncogene identified a subset of patients with poor prognosis, especially if the axillary lymph nodes show evidence of disease. It has also been shown that patients who express the C/erbB/2 also show a better response to adjuvant chemotherapy.

8. P53 - Expression of P53 protein or accumulation of it has been said to correlate with reduced patient survival. However, in patients who are node-negative, the accumulation of P53 was not a reliable prognostic marker.

9. BCL/2 - There is a relationship between BCL/2 protein expression and long-term survival in breast cancer patients. BCL/2 also correlates with estrogen receptor status.

10. Degree of angiogenesis - Recently a very interesting observation has been made that invasive cancers have prominent blood vessel component in their surrounding area, therefore they behave in a more aggressive fashion. Attempts are being made to quantitate the number of vessels that are present and to try and correlate these features as they relate to prognosis.

11. Cathepsin D and stromelysin - Presence of enzymes such as which, are involved in tumor invasion.

12. Extensive edema, multiple nodules in the skin - These are poor-prognostic signs. As well as spread to the chest wall, spread to internal mammary nodes, supraclavicular metastases, inflammatory carcinoma and distal metastases.

13. Factor of pregnancy - There is agreement that cancer of the breast which occurs during pregnancy or lactation has an overall poorer prognosis.

14. The presence or absence of invasiveness - This is the single most important prognostic determinator of breast cancer. In situ carcinomas are 100% curable with mastectomy. In ductal tumors that are in situ and also invasive there is a relationship between the proportion of the invasive component and the probability of spread to the lymph nodes.

Staging

Staging hopes to define the extent of disease and thus also helps to design the treatment for a particular stage. There are two types of staging:

1. Clinical staging

This includes examination of the breast by palpating or feeling the mass, examination of the skin, chest wall and armpit and neck for enlarged lymph nodes. Mammogram should be reviewed at this time also, as well as a tissue biopsy for a diagnosis of cancer. The amount of tissue examined for clinical staging is less than that needed for pathologic staging.

2. Pathologic staging

This includes all the information obtained from the clinical staging, findings at surgery and findings from pathologic examination of the tissue.

The primary tumor lies in the breast and is designated as T size and it can vary from T_x when size of the tumor cannot be assessed. T_0 = no evidence of tumor, T is in situ carcinoma, T_1 = size of tumor up to 2.0 cm. or less, T_2 = size of tumor 2.0 cm. to 5.0 cm., T_3 = size of tumor greater than 5.0 cm., T_4 = tumor of any size but involving the chest wall or skin.

Regional lymph nodes: Nx = when nodes cannot be assessed, N_0 = no regional lymph nodes, N_1 = metastases to moveable lymph nodes in the same armpit where the breast cancer is, N_2 = spread to lymph nodes fixed to one another, N_3 = metastases or spread to internal mammary lymph nodes on the same side.

Pathologic classification pN of regional lymph node involvement includes number and size of lymph nodes involved. All this information is important because it effects the behavior and natural history of the tumor.

Distant metastases or spread M_x. M_x = distant metastases cannot be assessed, M_0 = when there is no distant spread, M_1 = distant spread including spread to nodes above the collarbone.

Stage grouping

Stage O	Stage 1	Stage 2A	Stage 2B	Stage 3A	Stage 3B	Stage 4
Tis N_0 M_0	T_1 N_0 M_0	T_0 N_1 M_0	T_2 N_1 M_0	T_0 N_2 M_0	T_4, any N, M_0 ,	any T, any N, M_1
		T_1 N_0 M_0	T_3 N_0 M_0	T_1 N_2 M_0	any T, N_3 M_0	
		T_2 N_0 M_0		T_2 N_2 M_0		
				T_3 N_1 M_0		
				T_3 N_2 M_0		

Therapy

Current treatment of breast cancer includes:

1. Mastectomy
2. Lumpectomy with or without lymph node dissection
3. Post-op radiation
4. Chemotherapy

Surgical therapy There is a wide variety of options including radical mastectomy, partial mastectomy, that is, either a lumpectomy or segmentectomy, total simple mastectomy and modified radical mastectomy.

Chapter 14
PRIMARY CARE
PHYSICIAN'S ROLE IN MANAGEMENT
OF BREAST DISEASE

I went to my doctors and asked their advice
He's handsome, she's charming, they're both very nice.
But I'm thirty five and they still call me laddie;
(I guess it's because they're my mommy and daddy.)

In this discussion, the term "primary care physician" is used to include that physician whom the woman sees on a regular basis for her routine examinations. This may be her general practitioner, family practice physician or gynecologist, or in some cases, her oncologist.

Since these physicians usually know the patient well, they are the "first line" of information and treatment for most women with questions about their breasts. Recognizably, most problems will not be about cancer, but about developmental problems, problems related to childbirth and benign diseases. But it is understood that most women will receive a great deal of information from her primary care physician during her annual physical or gynecological examination. A primary care physician who does not carefully listen to questions and carefully examine the breasts is setting his/her patient and himself/herself up for disaster. The expectations of the public are such that these examinations must not only be done regularly but must be done seriously because of the high level of concern for early diagnosis if a patient has breast cancer.

The primary physician is usually the one responsible for advising the patient regarding the correct path to take on the diagnostic pathway, and therefore it is inherent upon this physician to be up-to-date in modern breast care management. For this reason we encourage continual updating in breast care through the guidance of the Comprehensive Breast Care Center, especially with regard to the ever-changing field of breast cancer management. The most conscientious primary physicians are frequently at the Breast Tumor Boards, and I can tell you that their patient management regarding breast disease is first rate.

The primary care physician will be able to advise his patient about the myriad of changes occurring in the course of a normal pregnancy and delivery, and answer the questions you have about breast engorgement, lactation, and nursing. The younger women will have concerns about rubbery round breast masses which are usually benign fibroadenomas and require no special attention unless they become large or symptomatic. The women with fibrocystic disease will be reassured by the skilled physician who can occasionally needle aspirate the cysts or refer her to the appropriate specialist. The patient can be counseled about the effects of caffeine on the breasts in exaggerating the problems of fibrocystic disease, and advise about stopping all caffeine for a month trial to see the effects. Caffeine is found in regular coffee, tea, many soft drinks, and sadly, also in chocolate. The fibrocystic disease can frequently cause very painful breasts, and the woman must decide whether she can live without her caffeine "fix". In severe cases of fibrocystic disease, some physicians will prescribe a drug called Danocrine which will significantly decrease the symptomatology, and often make most of the cysts disappear. There are some occasional unpleasant side effects, and these must be discussed with the patient before starting this medication.

Breast infections, or mastitis can occur in the lactating breast more frequently than in the "normal" breast, and usually responds to antibiotics. Women usually present with a painful, warm, tender breast, and this usually clears up in a few days on appropriate treatment. Rarely an abscess will develop which will need surgical intervention as described elsewhere.

The family physician will set the stage for the young woman entering into her thirties and forties by encouraging and instructing her in breast self-examination, and advising her to start yearly screening mammograms at age forty. There is controversy about this, however, and many new reports recommend not starting the routine mammographic studies until the patient is fifty. I personally have continued to recommend my patients and my primary care physician colleagues to continue with yearly screening from age forty onward until further data can answer the question more definitively. Patients with strong family histories or genetic propensity to breast cancer may even be recommended for mammograms in their thirties, although not on a yearly basis.

The family physician will be the best individual to counsel the patient on the value of good diet, birth control pills, exercise, and alcohol consumption, all of which are covered in different areas of this book.

Chapter 15
RADIOLOGY
AND BREAST DISEASE

Conrad Roentgen, in a daze,
Discovered some strange electrical rays.
And poised between O and X (hugs and kisses),
He chose the X, for he loved his missus.

So X rays were born, and we use 'em in tests
To see women's features, especially breasts.
But had he been more into hugging that day,
We'd probably be calling it now, the O ray.

The Radiologist is a physician trained in the use of X-rays and other similar forms of energy for the diagnosis and sometimes for the treatment of disease. Much like the pathologists, these physicians are often not seen by patients or have a very limited interaction with them. When invasive procedures such as angiograms or intestinal x-rays are performed, you may meet the radiologists briefly and when Breast Core Biopsies or needle localizations are done, their presence will be seen and felt but in general you don't get to talk much with them, and it is the rare radiologist who will put your x-rays in front of you and describe the findings. They usually interact directly with your physician by describing their findings, and often recommending further studies.

In today's world of medicine, patients demand more interaction with their physicians and again, we are fortunate in our Breast Center to have a physician who will take time out to speak at public forums and on a one-to-one basis with patients about their radiographical findings, and the patients greatly appreciate this interaction. Radiologists, Dr. David Cassidy and Dr. Stephen Simon, in addition to their work as diagnostic general radiologists, have become experts in radiology of the breast, and have become invaluable participants in the comprehensive breast program. Who better than they can I call upon to tell you about the field of medicine which has blossomed in our center under their expertise and enthusiasm?

THE HISTORY OF MAMMOGRAPHY

The radiographic examination of the breasts began within 20 years of the discovery of the x-ray by Roentgen. The first images were performed on mastectomy specimens. In the 1920's, patients with obvious breast abnormalities were examined with existing conventional x-ray equipment in an attempt to diagnose various breast diseases. Radiologists described various findings in normal breasts at different ages, as well as in pregnancy and various inflammatory conditions of the breast. In 1930's, the first large series of patients was reported in the United States with better than 90% accuracy in distinguishing benign versus malignant disease in preoperative symptomatic patients. However, this degree of accuracy was not consistently reproducible in subsequent studies, probably due to the lack of attention to image quality details, and that scientific interest in diagnostic mammography was limited until the 1950's.

Improvements occurred by the development of techniques of compression and proper exposure to all parts of the breast. The first dedicated mammographic x-ray machines were designed. Reports in the literature described the finding of microcalcification in the diagnosis of breast cancer which was important for the eventual use of mammography for screening in asymptomatic patients.

In the 1960's, there was further evolution of improvement in quality by the development of special x-ray generators, mammographic x-ray film, and unique positioning techniques. Over 50 otherwise occult cancers were reported in one large study. By 1965, it was established that the techniques of mammography could be standardized and learned by radiologists and technologists. Acceptable quality mammograms were reproducible. Differentiation could be made between benign and malignant diseases, and screening of asymptomatic patients was possible.

In the 1970's, further efforts were made to improve image quality while reducing radiation exposure to the patient. The developments included the use of automatic exposure timing, special x-ray tubes with microfocal spots, so-called rare earth screens and faster film. Proper film processing was also emphasized.

Separately, xeromammography was introduced with superior image quality and lower radiation dosage than existing screen-film systems. Xeromammography was advocated for its ease of detection of calcifications and spiculated masses. However, by the late 1980's, screen-film systems underwent further improvement with additional reduction in radiation exposure. That fact combined with the maintenance difficulties of the xeromammographic units resulted in the discontinued use and production by the Xerox company.

ACCREDITED MAMMOGRAPHY

The current state of mammography has been impacted greatly by the accreditation process. While much of the progress had been made in the 1970's and early 1980's to improve quality and decrease radiation exposure, there remained a wide variation in these factors among mammography units. When the American Cancer Society (ACS) began its national low cost screening program in 1987, there needed to be assurance that mammographic facilities met certain standards. In addressing this need, the American College of Radiology (ACR) began the voluntary ACR Mammography Accreditation Program. In the next seven years, approximately 2/3 of the mammography units in the United States had been accredited by this program. When Medicare reimbursement was approved for screening mammography, the federal government (HCFA) began to impose quality assurance regulations on facilities providing service to Medicare patients. These were very similar to those of the ACR program. Federal and state inspectors enforced regulations involving qualification of personnel, the volume of studies, processor performance, and documentation of quality control. Phantom assessment was made for image quality and radiation dosage. Clinical images were evaluated for positioning, contrast, motion, compression, labeling, and other factors. In 1992, the first Mammography Quality Standards Act (MQSA) became law and required all mammography facilities to be accredited regardless of their mix of Medicare and private patients for both screening and diagnostic procedure. Now the Food and Drug Administration (FDA) has the responsibility for determining that only accredited facilities be allowed to perform mammographic services.

BREAST BIOPSIES

Patients that are screened for breast cancer by mammography have by definition no clinical indication of benign or malignant disease. In spite of the highest quality images and interpretation, the findings are purely radiographic in nature, and while some are highly suspicious for malignancy, the majority are indeterminate in nature, and most of these turn out to be benign. If all of these patients were subjected to open surgical biopsy, the costs and risks involved considering the largely benign results would be unacceptable. For these reasons, various image guided methods of nonsurgical biopsy were developed and evolved. Surgeons and other clinicians have used fine needle aspiration (FNA) for several decades to provide histologic diagnosis of palpable breast masses. Initially, it was logical for radiologists to develop techniques for using fine needle aspiration to evaluate nonpalpable lesions detectable only by screening mammography. FNA is limited by the fact that only individual cells are obtained. These are often insufficient in number and fragile. The precision of needle placement is critical and the specific skills required for accurate diagnosis is not uniformly available in pathology departments.

For these reasons, large core biopsy systems guided by dedicated stereotactic x-ray equipment or ultrasound were developed. The size of core biopsy specimens as determined by the size of the needle progressed from 18 to 14 to 11 gauge. With the diameter of an 11-gauge needle, it became feasible to introduce tiny clips through the bore of the needle. This is required for later localization of the biopsy site in case the entire radiographic finding was removed by the needle biopsy procedure.

The specimens obtained by large core needle biopsy are superior to those obtained by FNA. They are stable, and easily preserved, and transported to the pathology department where a diagnosis is made with accuracy by conventional surgical pathology methods. Specimen radiographs are used to localize the microcalcification within the array of core specimens obtained, and immediate post-biopsy radiograph documents the removal of some or all of the suspicious findings, and the placement of the localization clip.

ULTRASOUND

Breast ultrasound uses sound waves to accomplish two main tasks: (1) to locate lesions within the breast, and (2) to characterize the composition of the lesions that are found. Every hearing person is familiar with sound waves, of course, since every noise we hear is composed of them. The major difference between audible sound and ultrasound is that ultrasound uses frequencies that are higher than humans are able to hear.

Attempts to use sound waves for locating objects date to at least the early part of the 20th century. After the Titanic sank in the North Atlantic in 1912, sound waves were utilized to try to find the ship on the ocean floor. It was not until World War II that a practical manner for using sound waves was developed with the invention of sonar (Sound Navigation Ranging).

After the war, the technology developed for sonar was adapted for medical applications. The first medical ultrasound patients had to be immersed in a vat of water, nearly duplicating a sonar scan in the ocean One "static" picture was produced on every pass the machine made. Since then, the advances in ultrasound instrumentation have been phenomenal. Today, a small amount of water-based gel is all that is needed between the scan head and the patient, and the images are updated continuously, i.e. they are "real-time".

Ultrasound is a very safe modality, with no serious biological effects having been found. This is particularly demonstrated by ultrasound's use in obstetrics, as the fetus is very sensitive to any injury. However, ultrasound has been used since 1958 to evaluate millions of pregnancies, and no ill effects have been shown.

Ultrasound locates an object in the same manner as a submarine's sonar. A short pulse of sound is sent out which bounces off an object and returns as an echo. The echo returns in a short time for close objects, and a long time for distant objects. By observing how long it took for the echo to return, the machine can precisely localize where the visualized object is.

Ultrasound characterizes the composition of what it sees by acoustic impedance, which is related to its density. A cyst, being fluid-filled, is much less dense than the surrounding tissue, and can be very easily identified. A solid nodule, though surrounded by solid tissue, is likely to be composed of different material than the tissue in its immediate vicinity, and therefore can be differentiated as well.

Because of its sensitivity in picking up both cystic and solid lesions, breast ultrasound was once touted as a replacement for mammography. Unfortunately, breast ultrasound, when used as a screening tool, picks up many benign conditions that can't be evaluated by ultrasound alone. However, when used in conjunction with mammography, ultrasound becomes a powerful tool.

Although mammography is the best modality available for breast imaging, there are nodules sometimes found which cannot be placed in definitely benign or definitely malignant categories by mammography alone. Ultrasound is an important adjunctive procedure in these cases.

Breast cysts are found in many women, but are almost universally benign. If a nodule seen on mammography is demonstrated to be a cyst by ultrasound, no further work-up is usually necessary.

However, a nodule that is found to be solid by ultrasound may be benign or malignant. There are criteria that help classify nodules as one or the other, such as shape, contour, and orientation. This information, coupled with the findings on mammography, help the radiologist decide what the next course of action should be.

Ultrasound is also used for a few specialized cases, such as palpable abnormalities that are obscured by overlying tissue on mammography. When used in this directed manner, ultrasound provides valuable information for a complete diagnostic evaluation.

Thermography

Breast cancer not only produces a mass of tumor cells; it also provokes changes in the surrounding tissues. One of the most important of these changes is the production of new blood vessels. Some researchers have used thermography in an effort to find cancers by this physiologic change in the breast.

Thermography utilizes a scanner that measures infrared radiation emitted by the body to create an image that maps out body temperature. Theoretically, cancers should be "hotter" than the surrounding breast because of the increased number of blood vessels. Unfortunately, the same pattern can be generated in breasts that do not have cancer. As such, thermography has not been found to be specific enough for diagnostic purposes at this time.

MRI

MRI (Magnetic Resonance Imaging) uses magnetic fields to produce cross-sectional images of the body. No X-rays or radioactive materials are used, and no harmful biologic effects have been found.

Current breast MRI research is focused on producing an anatomic picture that also demonstrates the physiologic changes that occur with breast cancer. This involves the injection of a contrast agent which enhances, or "lights up" cancers because of their increased vascularity. Other variables also have to be considered such as the appearance of the lesion, and the amount and pattern of enhancement. In practical use, breast MRI can be extremely difficult to interpret, so it is still classified as experimental at this time. The manner in which MRI images are acquired can be manipulated, though, and so research to refine the procedure further is continuing.

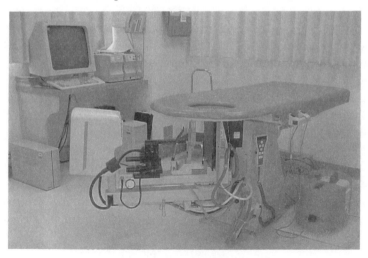

Figure 38. CORE BIOPSY TABLE.

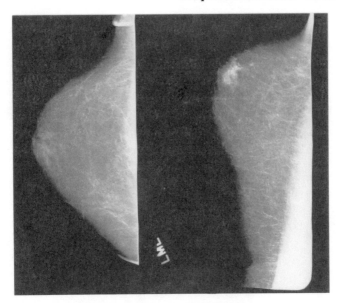

Figure 39. NORMAL MAMMOGRAM.

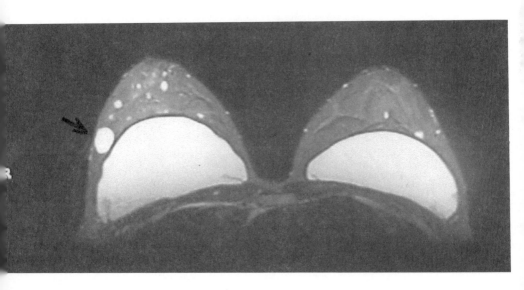

Figure 40. FIBROCYSTIC DISEASE IN IMPLANTS.

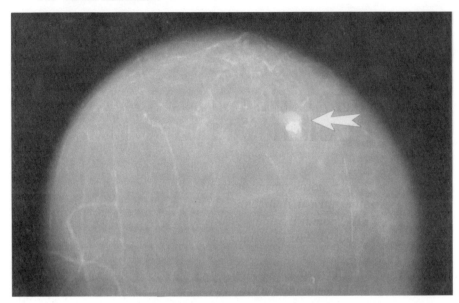

Figure 41. CALCIFIED FIBROADENOMA.

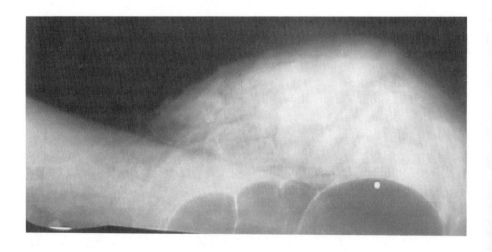

Figure 42. BIG LIPOMAS BEHIND THE BREAST.

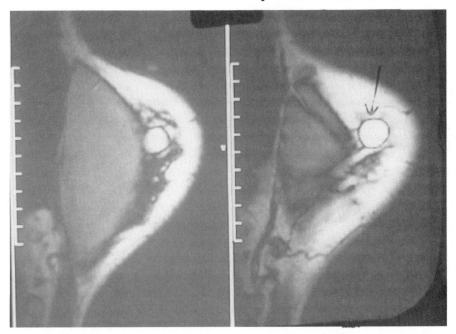

Figure 43. A LARGE CYST WITH BREAST IMPLANT.

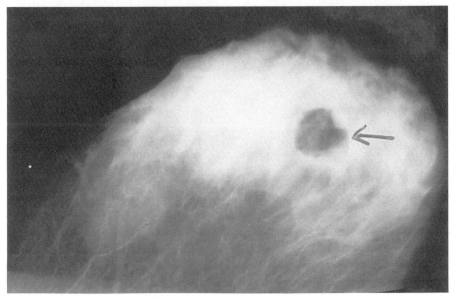

Figure 44. CYST OF A BREAST.

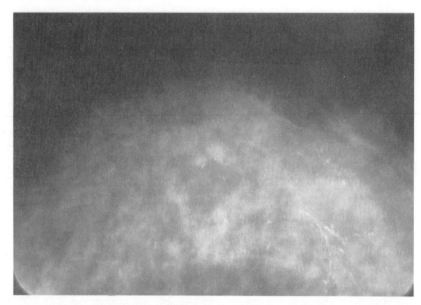

Figure 45. MICRO CALCIFICATIONS.

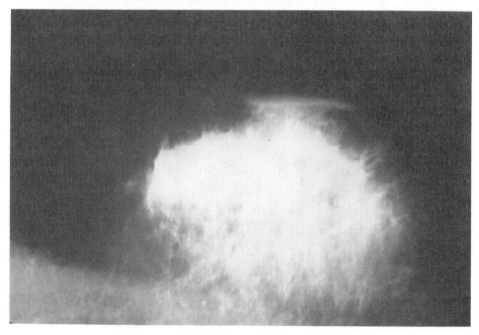

Figure 46. CANCER OF THE BREAST.

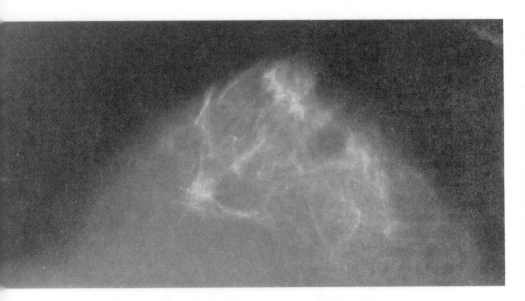

Figure 47. ANOTHER CANCER OF THE BREAST.

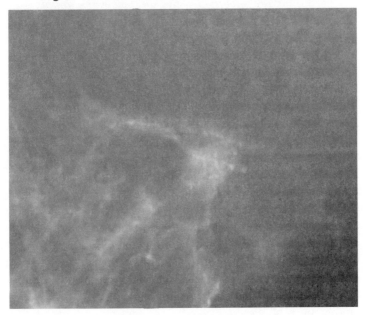

Figure 48. MAGNIFIED VIEW.

Chapter 16
GENETICS AND CANCER

Genes, genes, we're genetic machines
They control all our cells from our start thru our teens.
They cause us to grow eyes, hair, hemorrhoids, and spleens,
And everyone has 'em from bums up to queens.

Now it seems, we are told, that some bad ones cause cancer,
Just give us some cells, and we'll give you the answer.
BRCA one and two can cause breast tumors,
I heard it on fact, it's not just from rumors.

And that DNA coil you've heard so much about
Is what we're concerned with that causes the doubt.
So you need to be tested, if at a great risk
And counseled and checked on a Gail model disc.

And then we'll advise you, in words plain and simple
To say to your daughter, who's thirty with dimples:
"Do self exams, mammograms, and be well aware,
Your genes may cause cancer, and better beware".

NEW CENTURY, NEW WORDS, NEW RISKS, NEW PRECAUTIONS

For several years, I have been privileged to work with medical oncologist, Dr. Lalita Pandit. In recent years, she has taken a special interest in the field of medical genetics, and has received special training in the diagnosis and treatment of cancers based on genetic abnormalities. It is a relatively new field which will grow by leaps and bounds in the coming years as we understand more about the etiologies of cancer. Dr. Pandit is also involved now with a risk assessment program which has been started at the Center For Breast Care to evaluate each woman's risk for developing breast cancer, and she frequently lectures to physicians and the general public on this fascinating new area of medicine. I have written this chapter with her to explain to you concisely and understandably what is otherwise a very complex and challenging field.

Genetic counseling based on genetic evaluation is coming of age, and you and your physician better be aware of it. The comprehensive breast care program should include this in their overall evaluation to enable you to better understand breast disease.

So what is a gene? In our book, we are not considering something which is blue and worn by teenagers, hippies, cowboys, and some actresses. In simplest terms, a gene is a unit of hereditary information found in specific areas of a threadlike microscopic structure in all cells of our body called the chromosome. I'm not going to get more specific about this than to tell you that most humans have 46 chromosomes arranged in 23 pairs. These chromosomes are made up of that oft written about substance called DNA (deoxyribonucleic acid – say it four times fast). The entire field of genetics is built around these structures, and needless to say, becomes quite complex and esoteric. For our purposes, it is important to recognize that scientists are now able to identify and categorize genes as to function and importance. When there are abnormalities in certain genes or the presence or absence of certain genes, this can be traced to changes in the development of the human body and most recently associated with increased risk and tendency to form cancer in certain individuals.

Recent advances in technology and laboratory research have led to the association of genetic alterations with specific cancers. Although a majority of cancers cannot be predicted by genes at this time, there are a few defined syndromes (clusters of cancers in a family or a person) which are related to genetic changes and definitive inheritance patterns (you get it from one or both your parents like hair color, facial features, etc.), e.g., the unusual Li Fraumeni syndrome-- no, I won't tell you what it is.

The usual risks for developing breast cancer have been discussed elsewhere, but in review, they are:

1. Increasing age
2. Family history of breast cancer
3. Starting menstrual periods at an early age (nine or ten years old)
4. Late menopause (into the fifties)
5. Estrogen use
6. Dietary factors, especially alcohol.

A common thread may be the constant exposure of the breasts to estrogen, longer in women who menstruate over more years About 70-80% of breast cancers are sporadic (meaning we're still too dumb to know why), 15-20% occur in family clusters, and only 5-10% are hereditary.

The most well known genes identified as contributing to hereditary susceptibility to breast cancer are BRCA1 and BRCA2. Features that indicate increased likelihood of having BRCA mutations (changes in genes) are:

1. Multiple cases of early onset breast cancer and a history of ovarian cancers in a family
2. Breast and ovarian cancer in the same patient
3. Bilateral breast cancer
4. Male breast cancer
5. Ashkenazi Jewish heritage (Statistics indicate the highest incidence of BRCA1 and BRCA2 in this group).

The benefits of BRCA testing are in identifying high risk individuals and non-carriers (non-high risk individuals) in a family with known mutations. It also allows early detection followed by prevention strategies and may relieve anxiety.

When BRCA1 testing is positive in a patient, chances of developing breast cancer varies from 50-85% and that of ovarian cancer ranges between 15-45%. When breast cancer is diagnosed before age 40, the risk of being a carrier and having a mutation in BRCA1 ranges from 7-53%, depending on the number of first degree (close) relatives with breast cancer and their age. In women diagnosed with breast cancer after 40, the risk ranges from 4-15%. But regardless of the age at the time of diagnosis, a first degree relative with ovarian cancer indicates a 42% risk of carrying a mutation in BRCA1 (Wooster et al 1995).

BRCA2 gene, which is found on a different chromosome, account for 45% of familial breast cancers. A more important fact about the BRCA2 is its association with male breast cancer and prostate cancer.

Even when the BRCA test is negative in a family with breast cancer patients, there is a risk of unidentified familial genetic changes. In these cases, genetic counseling provides a very important role on generating a specific and individualized risk management. Aggressive screening in immediate family members of breast cancer patients should always be the norm. A recent well-publicized study in Breast Cancer Prevention in the United States offers a clinical trial for high risk patients who can take a drug called Tamoxifen. You can ask your oncologist about this and whether you should be one of the participants. A more radical approach for very high risk women, bilateral mastectomy, was studied in Europe but is yet to be studied significantly in the United States. Mastectomy, however, does still remain one of the options for breast cancer prevention in a very limited number of individuals, and only after comprehensive evaluation and psychosocial interaction.

Genetic Counseling is reasonable for any woman whose family has multiple cases of breast cancer. This counseling is done by trained specialists in conjunction with physicians and clinical psychologists. There are typically two categories for genetic testing, high risk and low risk, determined from responses by the patient to a detailed questionnaire. (See the discussion of the Gail Model). High risk patients typically undergo counseling and blood testing whereas low risk patients may only need counseling and no blood testing.

Although this relatively new field of gene testing sounds exciting, it does have its risks and limitations, since not all mutations are detected, and there is continued risk of sporadic cancers (where we don't yet know any genetic causation). We still need to weigh the advantages and disadvantages of this kind of testing because of the emotional, psychosocial consequences, and because of the economic consequences. Some states have protective laws preventing insurance companies from refusing health and life insurance to women who test positive for these cancer-affiliated genes. Sometimes what sounds and seems good and reasonable has more negative than positive consequences. So lastly, we must recognize that BRCA1 and BRCA2 mutations remain of restricted significance, and the exact cancer risk associated with these mutations is yet to be fully determined.

Another commonly known gene detected in breast cancer and which you may have read about or heard on TV is the HER-2/neu gene. Only a small percentage of patients with breast cancer express (have this on the blood test) the HER-2/neu gene, and we don't use this as a sign that you have an increased risk for breast cancer, as we do with BRCA. But the interest lies in the fact that we can now treat these patients with a new drug called Herceptin which actually targets against this gene!

In the future, genetics is going to play an increasing role in treatment modalities by offering drugs which can in some way alter your genetic propensity to develop a cancer. These modalities are presently investigational and soon you will hear more about drugs when they are taken from the laboratory to clinical trials on humans.

With our expanding knowledge about breast cancer etiology, there will, no doubt, be further discoveries about your body's ability to destroy cancer cells in their early stages, and genes will probably play an important role is this evaluation and therapy. We know that most of us have a continual production of abnormal cells and that our bodies are able to fight against these cells and destroy them. Apparently there is a point beyond which the body defenses are overwhelmed and cannot eliminate these "potential cancer cells". Hopefully in the future we will be able to boost the body's defense systems through immunological as well as other methods.

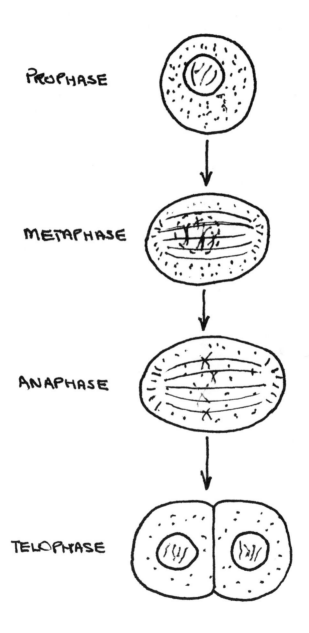

Figure 49. CELL IN MITOSIS.

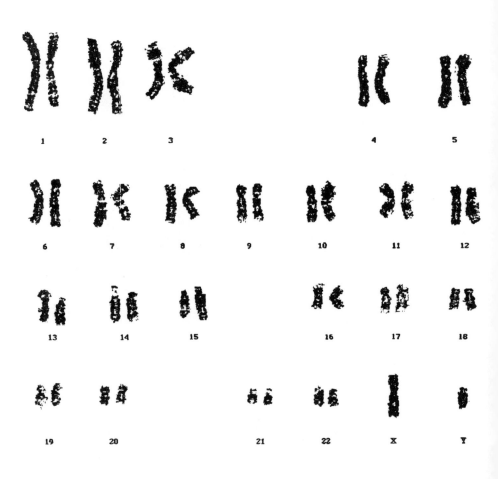

Figure 50. CHROMOSOMES.

Chapter 17
NURSING ADMINISTRATION
AND THE CANCER PATIENT

So you're the one who makes the rules,
One of the management, one of the ghouls.
You've never made a mistake or gaffe,
You see around comers like a large giraffe.

You're feared by everyone, loved by none
Have a countenance much like Attilla the Hun
But when there's a job that must be done,
I'll choose you, 'cause you're the best one.

If you're an administrator,
Gotta go, I'll see you later.

When we think of an administrator, we usually picture an individual behind a desk overseeing and directing an organization. In the comprehensive breast program, whether as an individual unit or part of a larger cancer center, the role of administrator is one of an individual wearing many hats. It is usually a complex position demanding a multiplicity of talents such as Nursing Specialist, Organization Person, Secretary, and "Multifactotum" or "Grand Poobah", who has a background in Oncology, Clinical Psychosocial ability with interviewing and directorial skills, Assertiveness, Financial Acuity, Computer Literacy, Tact, Political Savvy, and Chutzpah, to name a few.

This individual is often the glue that holds the diffuse parts of a large puzzle together and it is his or her ability that makes a Cancer Program succeed or fail. Look upon him or her as the Producer of a telecast melodrama who must join together the actors, directors, scenery crew, electricians, stagehands, costume designers and bankers to make the show a success financially and to please the audience. One weak link can impact the whole chain of events and it all falls back into that one person's lap. So it takes a person with past experience to be able to foresee and anticipate the problems and solve them rapidly.

So, why do we discuss this in a book about Comprehensive Breast Care? First, to let you know why finding a good program may be difficult and to give you the background to understand what to look for and how to ask for it. Second, and perhaps more important in the long run, to let you have the opportunity, if you so desire, to become one of the responsible persons who works in the network and helps this administrative individual make the program a success. "What do I mean and how do you do it?" you may ask. Whether you are a professional health care provider or a housewife or a businesswoman, you will want to participate in your local Comprehensive Breast Center in some capacity. Making a strong community effort starts with you and you don't have to be Mrs. Rockefeller or Mrs. Vanderbilt to make your presence felt. This book has outlined numerous areas where the "lay" individual can contribute and this leads us to the Administrator of the program. If he or she is wise, doors will always be open to the community for participation in some aspect of the deliverance of this important aspect of breast health. Let me diverge for a moment with a parable from mythology.

Narcissus was supposed to have been the most beautiful of men When he died, all the Flowers of the fields wept; they said that they loved him very much because he was so beautiful. The Stream then asked the Flowers: "Was Narcissus beautiful?" The Flowers answered by saying: "Stream, surely you knew that he was beautiful. Narcissus came every morning to look at the reflection of himself in your waters. You could see how beautiful he was." Stream replied: "If I loved Narcissus, it was not because he was beautiful, but because when he looked at the reflection of himself in my waters, I could see the reflection of my waters in his eyes!"

So blah blah--what's that got to do with anything? Just that in participating in a community effort such as a cancer or breast health program in any capacity, will allow you to see a reflection of yourself in the eyes of the many adults and children you will be helping in some small way. And the joy and satisfaction you will reap from such an interaction will not be measured in dollars but "in the reflection of your waters in Narcissus' eyes". Get involved!

It can be productive and also enjoyable. In our Cancer Center, we have a number of outreach programs, among them a luncheon at a local museum with speakers and entertainment, and a yearly Gala with a dinner, and live and silent auctions with everything from theater tickets, artwork, trips to Hawaii and Europe, to baseballs and movie memorabilia signed by the stars--something for everyone.

Chapter 18
PSYCHOSOCIAL APPROACH
TO THE PATIENT WITH CANCER

Hey, what do you think, I'm stupid or crazy,
Just 'cause I'm stubborn and a little bit lazy?
Why should I seek out some therapist or shrink,
Now that I'm not feeling quite in the pink?

Things are a bit rough and I can't win the lottery,
And just 'cause I smashed all the glasses and pottery
Don't mean I got problems that I can't just handle
With a good glass of wine and a bell, book and candle.

Those shrinks and psychologists are for the nut cases
The gals that can't make it around all the bases.
The strong ones like me can take care of ourselves
We hide our emotions, put feelings on shelves.

So don't get sucked in by the clap trap and babble,
Just sit yourself down to a nice game of Scrabble
And take lots of pills and antidepressants,
And buy yourself all kinds of expensive presents.

And when the proverbial__hits the fan
And when you have leaped in the old frying pan
Remember its better to be stubborn and dumb
Than to find a solution, the right place to come.

So if you're like me and you like to just suffer
And the world all around's getting rougher and rougher,
Don't read this here chapter, its just for the birds
A whole lot of nonsense and flap doodle words!

We can look at a psychosocial program much the way a novice looks at a gentle rafting trip. Some look forward to it, some are unsure, and some won't go near it. The reasons for refusing the rafting trip can be as obstruse as "the water's too cold, I don't want to get wet"; "the raft will tip over and I can't swim"; and a number of other frequently unbased excuses. When you tell someone that when properly done the raft won't tip over, they won't listen, and when you tell them about the peace and relaxation and fun of the water experience, they may say they don't have the time or desire for this. If they've never done it, and you say: "Try it, you might be surprised and like it", you may get a response like, "My uncle Mort tried and didn't like it so I'm sure I won't either!".

We sometimes fear new things or things we don't understand or just don't like the sound of And like in a raft where there is a guide, some won't go near a psychosocial group where there is a "guide" because it means giving up a little control; others may say, "I don't need to talk in a group, I can read it all in a book!".

You can look up pictures of gentle rafting down the Bow River in Banff National Park in Alberta, Canada, but until you actually go there and experience it for yourself, you can't understand the beauty and the overall experience.

That's much like the psychosocial program. You can read about it until you're "blue in the face", but experiencing it is different. We know that your immune system may improve with the "cleansing" of your emotional being, but not by reading this book, watching a film or reading a work on self-help. It's the interaction with others with similar problems, with the guidance of a therapist, that makes it work.

Nevertheless, many of my patients refuse this service because of some preconditioned behavior. They think that they need to be in control, and the group scene will somehow make them lose control. The individual in the group actually has more control by facing her problems and resolving them. So don't close the door on this area of treatment, whether its for cancer or any other support group. Condemnation prior to examination is not only stupid, it's probably harmful in the long run.

So let us move on to hear from Ms. Lori Ash, Manager of Psychosocial Services at The Orange County Regional Cancer Center, a very experienced therapist who has dealt with all types of psychosocial problems in her professional life. We can look through her eyes at a strong psychosocial program which she has developed in Southern California; her experience can serve as a good example of what you should expect to find in any Comprehensive Cancer Center, and in a good center for breast care.

PSYCHOSOCIAL ISSUES AND CARE

For the past twenty years, I have had the opportunity to participate at many levels in the psychosocial spectrum of care regarding breast health concerns, both benign and malignant. Reflectively, it appears that breast health "issues" may begin for all of us as women at a very early age. This continuum spans across our lifetime, from early childhood and extending throughout each decade and into the new millennium. With continual development in the quest for expanded knowledge and improvement in the areas of breast health, diagnostic techniques, and breast cancer treatments, we as women have had an enormous amount of information throughout our lifetime regarding these issues. The many systems in our life which have "input" into this area may include: The media, newspaper articles, magazines, television, the Internet, our doctors, medical staff, parents, family members, friends, co-workers, counselors and "others".

Basically, there is a tremendous amount of breast health/cancer information as a part of our everyday life. It is everywhere For women concerned about breast health issues as well as women who have been diagnosed with breast cancer, this information can oftentimes be extremely helpful, somewhat confusing or quite stressful. Perhaps you are one of these women and can identify with these feelings. If so, you are definitely not alone!

To be available to focus on these concerns requires a beginning. The development of a pilot program at the Center for Breast Care (CBC) subsequently emerged---The Comprehensive Breast Exam Clinic. In addition to the regularly scheduled screening mammogram; the multidisciplinary team designed, implemented, and made available: Clinical breast exam by a physician, discussion of mammographic findings from the radiologist, education, prevention, nutritional guidelines, resources and supportive discussion. The Department of Psychosocial Services was asked to participate in the planning, implementation as well as the on-going review process of this program at the CBC. Embracing the emotional breast health fears and concerns that may "peak" at the time of mammography is vital in providing excellence of care. It is not unusual to hear participant comments at the CBC such as, "My best friend just found out she has breast cancer" or "Some of the women in my family have breast cancer and I worry that I may be at high risk". It seems that everyone knows someone who has been touched by a breast cancer diagnosis. Following the mammogram and radiologic findings, the Comprehensive Breast Exam Clinic "team" then meets with the patient. This includes a doctor, clinical social worker (or graduate social work intern), and a volunteer from the American Cancer Society (ACS) who is a breast cancer survivor and involved in Reach to Recovery. This overall program is outlined in another chapter.

The role of Psychosocial Services at the CBC is to provide the professional clinical social work component to this program. These include: Emotional support for all women who participate in the program (focusing on the special needs of those with "suspicious" or "abnormal" findings), normalizing feelings and concerns, identification and provision of vital resources, encouraging participants to ask "all" their questions, to acknowledge and promote cultural sensitivity, and to be available for follow-up services as indicated.

Additionally, an educational/informational packet has been collaboratively developed and is provided to each woman who participates in this comprehensive screening. An opportunity to view a breast self-exam video with the ACS volunteer present to address questions is also furnished (video available in English, Vietnamese, Chinese, and Spanish). Understandably, women are certainly concerned regarding breast cancer. This is especially true due to the high incidence in Orange County. Assisting women to more fully understand breast changes, encouraging regular mammograms, providing the training video in breast self-exam (BSE) techniques coupled with the importance of compliance, and stressing the importance of scheduling regular clinical breast exams is achieved through education, information, increased awareness, advocacy and support.

In addition to the services provided at the CBC, Psychosocial Services are available for women as well as their family members and loved ones in the form of supportive counseling. This continuum of care spans from the time of breast biopsy, following diagnosis, when a malignancy is discovered, and at every stage of the breast cancer experience. For any woman who has traveled this path, it can oftentimes seem as if life has become a roller coaster ride (and who or what is now in control?). Finding help and finding hope are crucial factors in the road to recovery. The "impact" as well as the "implications" following a breast cancer diagnosis can be very similar or at times as different as we are to one another. It is very important to remember that there are no "right" or "wrong" ways to feel. We as human beings are born with a full "complement" of emotions, and cancer can certainly draw on many of these. The emotional responses may include but certainly are not limited to shock, denial, anger, anxiety, guilt, fear, bargaining, depression, sadness, and acceptance. These emotions follow no true predictable course for all women with breast cancer, and can occur singularly, in combination, and even "unexpectedly" over the course of the breast cancer journey.

The myriad of psychosocial aspects of breast cancer and treatment are understandably linked with emotional factors. In gathering information over the years from women with breast cancer, their family members and loved ones, I have compiled a list of psychosocial issues. Certainly this list is by no means complete, but is meant to be of assistance in promoting further understanding:

- Impact of diagnosis, treatment plan and choices, as well as prognosis issues
- Sharing the diagnosis with others (who, what to tell them, and when)
- Knowing "what" questions to ask the doctor
- Change in body image
- Self-esteem issues
- Dealing with potential side effects (short-term and long-term, i.e. hair loss or lymphedema)
- Relationship/Communication Issues

- Concern for the family and certainly the children
- Feelings of isolation, being alone, or "different" following diagnosis
- Challenges to the existing support network
- Lack of information regarding vital resources and programs
- Difficulty in learning a whole new "oncology" language
- Loss of control/prior level of decision making
- Increased financial concerns (potential or real)
- Medical insurance coverage issues
- Dealing with the issue of uncertainty
- Restricted ability to plan ahead

Short-term/Long-term goal disruption
- Cultural/spiritual/religious factors
- Compromised employment/vocational/educational pursuits
- Transportation difficulties
- The potential for increased fatigue
- Change in appetite/nutritional status
- Sleep disorders
- Role difficulties: Patient/Family Member/Loved Ones
- Sexuality/Intimacy Issues
- Fertility Issues
- Genetic Testing
- Defining or "redefining" hope
- Survivorship (Fears following completion of treatment and "reconnecting" with life)
- Concerns regarding recurrence
- Quality of Life Factors

In the clinical practice and treatment of women diagnosed with benign breast disease as well as those diagnosed with metastatic breast cancer, increased awareness and understanding of the array of psychosocial factors is tantamount to comprehensive care. It is also crucial in determining an individualized treatment plan. Throughout the breast cancer experience and at each stage of treatment, a reassessment and monitoring of these issues can be very beneficial, for the patient as well as the treatment team. Initial and on-going psychosocial assessments are available as a part of our oncology program. To assist in this process, the Department of Psychosocial Services have additionally developed an "easy reading" brochure which outlines the comprehensive psychosocial services available. It delineates the role, training, and function of the oncology social worker, and indicators for psychosocial referral. These brochures are available to medical staff as well as patients and their family members.

Provision of educational/informational/resource packets that have been collaboratively developed with ACS are available to all women who have been newly diagnosed with breast cancer. M a n y "systems" in a woman's life can certainly be impacted by a myriad of psychosocial concerns as well. In viewing ourselves through a bio-psycho-social-cultural-spiritual model, the thread that is woven throughout the breast cancer experience can touch many facets in our life. These include self, family, friends, colleagues, vocational, educational financial, spiritual/religious, and cultural. Oftentimes the emphasis is on the patient alone. But through this model and in your own lives, certainly a comprehensive approach to care must include sensitivity to and services focused on aspects of each woman's own system. At the Orange County Regional Cancer Center, the vision which remains constant is a direct focus on excellence of care, including a commitment to the provision of targeted professional, comprehensive psychosocial services. These are available not only to the woman with breast cancer, but also to her "system" as well. In addition to the supportive counseling previously described, cancer support groups are also provided. They have been designed from a psycho-educational model that includes expert speakers in selected fields of oncology as well as supportive discussion meetings. All current cancer support groups are outlined and listed below to benefit the person who is reading this chapter. In providing this to you, we are hopeful that you have an understanding and utilizing the multidisciplinary treatment team (we are here to help you) in,

- Reviewing prior coping skills, the strengths within us, and attempting to live "with" cancer, one day at a time.
- Accessing the issue of hope (which is a prescription with absolutely no side effects!)

As we enter the new millennium, breast health concerns will certainly continue. It is anticipated that we can anticipate further progress to focus on such areas, as those of prevention, education, research, treatment, and quality of life studies. Embracing vital psychosocial issues and concerns to parallel this growth remains an essential priority. It also reflects a dedicated partnership. We invite all of you to join us as we venture forward toward this goal.

Chapter 19
DIET AND NUTRITION

They say that there's a little creature living in your brain
That loves to eat dark chocolate and purple candy cane
That little creature is yourself and has no sense of judgment
Its appetite is awesome and its choice of food is sludgement.

I know what's good and bad for me, I learned it as a child
But that small creature always wins and drives me nearly wild.
Now, if I had my druthers, I would make him go away,
I'd give an ultimatum...for a departing day.

I tried to solve the problem
But I'm feeling rather glum,
He said he'd leave tomorrow
But tomorrow never comes.

All you have to do is drive down Main Street, America to be faced with a myriad of stores selling all types of dietary supplements claiming cures for this and that. The only thing different from the covered wagon huxters of one hundred years ago is the packaging and slicker marketing techniques. Newspapers and magazines are ripe with all types of diets and supplements appealing to your sense of guilt and desire for well being. The general public spends hundreds of millions of dollars on these so-called panaceas. But we must acknowledge that mixed in with the cozenage, obfuscation, and hocus-pocus, there is also a great deal of valuable dietary information which we are fortunate to have gleaned from this morass of nonsense.

Jean French is a registered dietician. She is The One you turn to when you have questions about diet, supplements and the relative value of abstruse nostrums and oil-of-witches'-tooth She's knowledgeable and not fooled by slick advertising and unsubstantiated cure-alls. For her expertise, both her wisdom with words and her words of wisdom on this subject, I am very grateful. So here is Jean French telling you about Nutrition:

YOUR DIET, FRIEND OR FOE!

The idea that our diet may influence how the body functions is well understood by most Americans. But, for the majority of us, it is not translated into behavior by what we actually stick in our mouth. Most of us reach for that megavitamin that promises extra energy, youth and health to balance out the "Value Meal" just consumed at the local fast food joint. It is so much easier to pop a pill or mix a "shake" than to plan a meal from "real food". Information from the newspaper, TV or books and magazines seems to conflict and changes from week to week. The majority of women who are concerned about their diet and its' influence on their risk of breast cancer ask three basic questions:

1. Can my diet reduce my risk of breast cancer?
2. What should I eat and what should I avoid?
3. How do I incorporate the right foods into my diet?

1. Can My Diet Reduce My Risk of Breast Cancer?
As science began studying breast cancer and looked at different population groups, our "diet" became one of the environmental factors that was obviously different and may be the one factor or risk we might improve. Cancer begins by a few cells with changes in the DNA structure or blueprint that begins dividing improperly and continuing this process. It is the body's natural immune system that intervenes and stops the improper cell division or code. It is thought that certain foods inhibit this cell division or promote a desired cell death that stops the sequence of cell multiplication in the cancer process. By consuming certain foods that are believed to protect against cancer, a person may be improving the body's natural immune response. The problem begins with what our knowledge base is built on. The majority of what we know about our diet and its implications in the cancer process is built on observations or

association-type data. This information is just the beginning or the building block that further research is built on.

An example of this would be the previous belief that diets high in fat may increase a woman's risk of breast cancer. This hypothesis was developed from looking at different populations, determining the amount of fat that was consumed, and their associated breast cancer risk. When clinical trials were developed to confirm this hypothesis, much of the data was conflicting. Currently we are not quite so sure of fat intake and its implication on breast cancer. Most experts are beginning to look at the importance of maintaining a healthy body weight rather than just fat intake alone. Some studies have shown that excess body fat increases the estrogen level, especially in postmenopausal women. In the fat tissue, a hormone synthesizes estrogen from these fat stores, and it becomes the body's major source of estrogen after menopause. A rise in the estrogen level in a woman's body may increase the risk of breast cancer up to two times since breast cancer is thought to be a hormonally driven cancer.[1] [2]

Research showed that a recent increase in weight after menopause is associated with a concurrent rise in the risk of breast cancer in a woman. To combat this risk, the National Institute of Cancer recommends limiting weight gain to 11 pounds in the adult years.[3] In reality, healthy eating is a lifestyle that encompasses more than food but involves exercise. For a woman to experience the healthy lifestyle she desires, it must include exercise. Good nutrition and exercise dovetail together and become the building blocks for good health. Exercise does not have to be joining a gym, or buying an aerobic video but it does mean movement. Pick hobbies that involve movement such as gardening or biking. Join a group that walks or swims. Instead of taking your car to the car wash, do it yourself. Look for ways in your everyday life to increase your activity. But before starting any exercise program, discuss your plans with your physician.

2. What Should I Eat and What Should I Avoid?

All research emphasizes the importance for all Americans to increase their intake of fruits and vegetables in their diet. The recommendation from the American Institute of Cancer Research is to eat a variety of at least 5 or more servings of fruits and vegetables per day.[3] Fruits and vegetables are high in nutrients, yet low in calories and fat. They have naturally occurring vitamins and minerals that act as antioxidants. It is the antioxidant quality that is sought after to alter or stop the cancer process.

In our daily lives within our bodies are chemical reactions that produce a substance called "Free Radicals". A free radical is a chemical that when it interacts with other body tissues causes a break down in the body's normal function. Our body produces other chemicals whose purpose it is to stop the destructive interaction or neutralize the free radicals. This is exactly what antioxidants do. Fruits and vegetables also contain phytochemicals (phyto=plant) that also participate in the antioxidant process. Some phytochemicals such as lycopene found in tomatoes have stronger antioxidant qualities than the traditionally known antioxidants like beta-carotene. Other food items such as grains (wild rice, brown rice, millet, etc.), tuber-like plants (potatoes, plantains, yams, etc.) and legumes contain phytochemicals which are a part of the healthy diet in cancer prevention. Science in the past has tried to isolate nutrients and separate them from their natural environment. The isolated nutrient is sold alone or with other vitamins and minerals in the form of a pill or powder. In separate form, the chemical (whether a vitamin, mineral, or phytochemical) is not as useful as when put together. Research is quickly realizing that the pill antioxidant qualities are not the same as found in whole food. Vitamins, minerals and phytochemicals work together synergistically as a team to help the body perform its functions in an optimal manner. Some act as precursors and set the stage for a desired interaction, while others help the interaction or chemical reaction along. Currently, we do not know all the vitamin, mineral or plant chemicals that are needed in specific amounts to provide the best antioxidant protection. This is why a variety of different types of food are important.

Even though research on fat intake and it's impact on breast cancer is conflicting, it is still recommended to limit fat in the diet especially from animal origin.[3] By limiting fat, the tendency for a low calorie diet is improved and undesired weight gain may be controlled. One general recommendation is to limit red meat (beef and pork) to no more than 3 ounces per day. A 3-ounce serving is approximately the size of a deck of cards. Most Americans consume a larger portion than 3 ounces of meat at meal times. The emphasis for good protein source or low fat meat is more toward poultry and fish or even vegetarian entrees. The purpose in limiting red meat or reducing meat consumption is to reduce saturated fat intake. Saturated fat is found in food of animal origin such as meat, whole dairy products and vegetable fat like palm oil, coconut or palm kernel oil. Even margarine is considered a saturated fat because of the chemical process involved in making it. Medical science has documented for years the association of a high saturated fat intake and the increased risk for heart disease, but current research is showing a possible increase in the risk of breast cancer also.[4] The change in risk level may be from a higher calorie intake or possible insulin resistance associated with a high saturated fat diet. When a person's body is resistant to insulin, the body produces more insulin to overcome this resistance. One theory is that the increase of insulin in the blood may increase the hormone level and trigger the cancer process.[4]

In addition to the saturated fat content of the diet, some research associate a diet high in Omega-6 polyunsaturated fatty acids (n-6 PUFA) may increase a woman's cancer risk. This fatty acid is found in vegetable oil such as corn, safflower and other blends. Omega-3 fatty acid (n-3 PUFA) found in canola, peanut, olive, flaxseed and fish oils have a protective effect and may decrease cancer risk. The cell membrane, which is the body's first defense against cancer, is affected by what type of PUFA is consumed. In addition to changes in the cell membrane structure, the type of PUFA may stimulate or suppress the body's immune response.[5]

The one food which is the most controversial is soy. It was previously believed that a high intake of soy would be protective against breast cancer. Asian countries with a high intake of soy had a lower incidence of breast cancer than other countries with no or low soy intake. It is now thought other mechanisms such as increased physical activity, low fat or decreased red meat intake, a high vegetable diet alone or in combination, may be the reason for a lower incident. Soy foods have a phytochemical called genestein. This nutrient is structurally similar to tamoxifen, which is a chemotherapy drug used to fight breast cancer. Genestein can inhibit the body's acceptance of estrogen in the cell, and it was this mechanism that was thought to be protective. However, when the estrogen level is low, genestein can also act as a weak estrogen and may promote cancer in women diagnosed with breast cancer or in remission.[6] Certain research is looking at the phytochemical genestein (an isolated part of a food product) and its possible role in inhibiting cell growth or promotion of a desired cancer cell death called apoptosis. Just how this research is translated into diet recommendations is unclear.

Some studies show an increase in cell growth with genestein.[6,7,8] At this time, it is really unknown what the true effect soy has in its role in cancer prevention or in women diagnosed with breast cancer. Further research is needed to determine whether genestein in a food product will produce the same results as if taken separately as a supplement.

The intake of alcohol is associated with an increase in breast cancer risk. The major discrepancy lies in just how much is safe. One study showed a 40% increase with one drink a day (12-18 grams per day) over an average lifetime. The association of alcohol's effect and the breast cancer risk is stronger with postmenopausal women than premenopausal. Recent alcohol consumption contributes to a stronger risk of breast cancer while consumption prior to the age of 30 did not seem to affect a woman's risk. The type of beverage such as wine may not change a woman's risk possibly because of phenolic compounds which may have protective antioxidant qualities. However, beer and liquor may contain estrogen-like substances that may increase the breast cancer risk.[9] Before a woman decides to engage in alcohol consumption, she needs to evaluate her overall breast cancer risk and all potential side effects involved in alcohol consumption.

3. How Do I Incorporate The Right Foods Into My Diet?

Begin by increasing fruit and vegetable intake. Try to eat one fruit at every meal and for at least one snack. Add one to two servings of vegetables at lunch and dinner plus possibly one at snack time. One serving is usually:

* 1/2 cup cooked vegetables or fruit;
* 1 cup of raw vegetables
* A medium size fruit (apple or orange, etc.);
* 2 small fruits (apricots, plums)

Emphasize variety to obtain as many natural vitamins, minerals and antioxidants as possible. Try blends of different vegetables and sauté to a slightly crunchy consistency, then chill with a light dressing for a salad at lunch or a snack. Do not forget the traditional fresh vegetables with dip but be careful of the fat content in the dip. Choose low fat or fat free yogurt based dressings for dips. For additional preparation techniques or how to include an unusual fruit or vegetable in a meal, look at different ethnic foods. Observe the spices used, whether it's served hot or cold and the coordination of usual and not so familiar foods. Be adventurous and try new flavors and foods. The larger the variety to choose from improves the chances of meeting the 5 or more servings of fruit and vegetables recommended by the American Institute for Cancer Research. For a spicy fat free alternative for a salad dressing or potato topper, try salsa with a tablespoon of fat free sour cream.

Monitor fat intake by decreasing meat portion sizes. Limit portions to 2-3 ounces per serving and no more than 6 ounces of meat per day. A 2-ounce portion is approximately equal to one chicken leg or thigh, or a small hamburger patty from the traditional kid's meal served by fast food restaurants. The size and thickness of a deck of cards is approximately a 3-ounce portion or one half of a large chicken breast. Choose only lean mean, and choose a cooking method where the fat can drip off or away from the meat cut. Avoid cooking meat at high temperatures (i.e., broiled, grilled, seared or fried) which may produce heterocyclic amines. Avoid cooking meat in direct contact with flame (i.e., barbecuing, flame broiled or charbroiled) which produce polycyclic aromatic hydrocarbons. Both of these substances are known cancer-causing agents. Alternative methods of food preparation are to marinate the meat product first or precook the item in the microwave, and then grill or broil for flavor. Both alternative methods may reduce heterocyclic amine formation by 90 percent.[10] When fat is needed in food preparation, choose a monounsaturated fat such as canola or olive oil. When preparing a casserole dish, decrease the amount of meat stated in the recipe but improve the volume by adding additional grain, legumes or vegetables. Try a low fat vegetarian alternative but beware, not all-vegetarian entrees are healthy choices. Many of these can be high in fat. Purchase a vegetarian cookbook that emphasizes low fat cooking.

This will provide alternatives to the traditional meat-based meals and at the same time improve vegetable and fruit consumption. Add flavor to meals by using herbs and/or low sodium broths instead of butter, heavy gravies or sauces. Substitute nonfat evaporated milk for whole milk or cream in a sauce recipe. Choose nonfat or at least low fat (1% fat) dairy foods. Most importantly, read food labels. Don't assume a fat free product is always the best choice. Fat free foods are not necessarily calorie free and can promote weight gain. Take notice of the fat content per serving, the type of fat provided (saturated versus poly or monounsaturated), the calories per serving, and the recommended serving size or number of servings per package. For a low fat dessert or snack, try to limit the fat content to 3 grams and calories to no more that 200 per serving.

When baking, substitute unsweetened applesauce for up to one half of the fat content in a recipe. For chocolate recipes, try prune puree for part of the fat content. Instead of using frosting for a cake, top with fresh fruit slices or a fruit sauce sprinkled with powdered sugar for a low fat alternative. When baking cakes, cookies or muffins, substitute 2 egg whites for 1 whole egg for a nonfat, no cholesterol option or use 1/4 cup of egg substitute.

Don't forget to include grains and legumes in your diet which also contain phytochemicals. Traditionally grains are also high in fiber so remember to drink plenty of fluids when adding these foods to your diet. Substitute couscous, wild rice, millet, bulgar, kasha or barley for rice. Cookbooks can be your greatest source of inspiration. In casseroles, substitute 1/2 the required starch (ie rice, noodles, potatoes) with legumes such as lentils. Cook the legumes in a low sodium broth for extra flavor before adding to soup, casserole or side dish.

In Summary:
1. Maintain a healthy weight and increase your physical activity.
2. Consume 5 or more servings of fruit and vegetables a day.
3. Decrease fat intake. Emphasize monounsaturated fat and consume less saturated fat.
4. Increase fiber intake by incorporating whole grain, legumes and fresh fruit and vegetables into your diet.
5. Avoid alcohol.

Some helpful references for additional information on nutrition and it's impact on cancer:
- American Cancer Society
  1-800-227-2345
- American Institute of Cancer Research
  1-800-843-8114, Website: http://www.alcr.org
- American Dietetic Association
  1-800-366-1655, Website: http://www.eatright.org
- Eating Hints From U.S. Department of Health and Human Services 1-800-4 Cancer

NOTES

1. Cummings JH, Bingham SA. *Diet and the prevention of Cancer.* BMJ, 1998, 317 (12): 1636-40.
2. Kaas R, VanNoord PA, DenTonkelaar I, Peeter PHM, Riboli E., Grobbee DE. *Breast-Cancer incidence in relation to height, weight and body-fat distribution in the Dutch "DOM" cohort.* Int.J. Cancer, 1998; 76: 647-51.
3. American Institute for Cancer Research. *Food, nutrition and the prevention of cancer: A global perspective.* Washington DC: AICR, 1997.
4. Stoll BA. *Essential fatty acids, insulin resistance and breast cancer risk.* Nutrition and Cancer, 1998; 31 (1): 72-77.
5. Bagga D, Capone S, Want HJ, Heber D, Lill M, Chap L, Glaspy JA. *Dietary medication of Omega-3/Omega-6 polyunsaturated fatty acid ratios in patients with breast cancer.* Journal of the National Cancer Institute, 1997; 89 (15): 1123-31.
6. Verma SP, Goldin BR. *Effects of soy-derived isoflavonoids on the induced growth of MCF-7 cells by estrogenic environmental chemicals.* Nutrition and Cancer, 1998; 30 (3): 232-239.
7. Wang C, Kurzer MS. *Effect of phytoestrogens on DNA synthesis in MCF-7 cells in the presence of estradiol or growth factors.* Nutrition and Cancer, 1998; 31 (2): 90-100.
8. Sathyamoorthy N, Gilsforf JS, Wang TTY. *Differential effect of Genistein on Transforming Growth Factor B-1 expression in*

normal and malignant mammary epithelial cells. Anticancer Research, 1998; 18: 2449-2454.

9. Liongnecker MP, Newcomb PA, Mittendorf RJ, Greenburg ER, Clapp RW, Bogdan GF, Baron J, et al. *Risk of breast cancer in relation to lifetime alcohol consumption.* Journal of the National Cancer Institute, 1995; 87 (12): 923-29.

10. *American Institute for Cancer Research Newsletter.* Summer, 1999; 64: 4-5.

Chapter 20
CANCER OF THE BREAST AND CHEMOTHERAPY

Oncologists are Cancerophiles
They read it and write it and study it with smiles.
They work with the drugs that kill tumor cells,
(Some use incantations and old witches' spells!)

Their drugs have long names and they cost you high fees,
To treat every kind of disturbing disease.
And even if you don't want to praise 'em or tout 'em
It's hard for a patient to pull through without 'em.

The most difficult word for the practicing physician to relay to a patient with a breast problem is "Cancer". It denotes a disease, but it also connotes to most women "fear", "surgery", "chemotherapy", "suffering", "deformity", and "dying" The word itself has become a euphemism for all the fears and worries about health and patients and doctors alike have, in the past, shied away from its use. The literature is ripe with all the "almost cancer" words such as tumor, malignancy, growth, blight, curse, evil, trouble, etc., etc... But in today's world, we have made great progress in educating the public as well as physicians to the importance of facing each problem and dealing with it appropriately. Cancer, like TB, AIDS, and Diabetes Mellitus has come out of the closet of vagueness, ignorance, and inexpert expertise to the openness of knowledge, care, treatment and most of all, cure.

The diagnosis, once made, is followed by a comprehensive evaluation by the Tumor Board and the multiple members representing several subspecialties, offering a cohesive approach to treatment. We have covered the very extensive field of Cancer in several areas of this book--Pathology (describing the tissue cell changes and the types of cancer and staging), Radiology (discussing radiological diagnosis and core biopsy), and the many different possible Surgeries. We have discussed Radiation Therapy, Psychosocial support groups, and the Information Center. So now we must talk about the other word so maligned by the public–"Chemotherapy".

We immediately think of nausea, vomiting, hair loss, and suffering. The major nausea, vomiting, and sufferings are things of the past; we have very effective new drugs for controlling nausea and vomiting as well as medications for abnormal blood counts and infection. Remember, we are treating a disease which requires powerful medication to eradicate it completely or stem its growth. It is very strong medicine and thereby has strong side effects. While we can frequently eliminate or alleviate many of the side effects, some must be accepted and tolerated as an unfortunate but necessary "evil" such as temporary hair loss, appetite suppression, mild nausea and weakness.

So after all the comprehensive workup and the decisions made by the tumor board, the woman with breast cancer will often need chemotherapy. But first we should ask: "When don't we need chemotherapy?"

Obviously:

1. When there is No Cancer--some of the alternative treatments talk about treating "pre-cancer"--Hooey. Anti-cancer drugs are for cancer.
2. When the Cancer is Stage 0 or DCIS (ductal carcinoma in situ); many oncologists will not treat the patient except to place her on medication such as Tamoxifen.
3. When you don't want it!--Remember it's always your choice--- regardless of the wisdom or lack of wisdom behind your decision, you should either be satisfied with the treatment plan, seek a second opinion or seek other help!

In the remainder of this chapter, Dr. Glen Justice offers his wide range of experience with chemotherapy as a practicing private clinical oncologist and a teaching clinical professor at the USC Norris Cancer Center. He is a compassionate physician who always weighs the efficacy with the side effects before entering into this most serious area of patient care.

In understanding breast cancer and the importance and the role of chemotherapy, it is critical to understand some aspects of cancer itself. If one cuts oneself while shaving, the normal cell will multiply and divide 10 to 15 times, and then it will stop its cell division. The normal cell will be orderly and not violate its boundaries. Cancer cells differ in two fundamental ways. The first characteristic of cancer cells is that the cancer cell can divide and multiply indefinitely. It is truly uncontrolled growth or cell proliferation. The second characteristic of cancer cells is the ability (unlike normal cells) to spread to other organs via blood vessels and then grow in the other organs. This tendency to spread to other organs, such as the lung, liver, and bone, is the concept of metastases. In the case of breast cancer, it tends to spread to local lymph nodes, and then through the blood vessels, to the bone, lung and liver. Chemotherapy are medications that preferentially kill the more fragile and delicate cancer cell as compared to the more hardy normal cell, and thereby increase the cure rates in women with breast cancer. It is not unreasonable that chemotherapy can increase cure rates and survival in breast cancer, for these same drugs have dramatically increased the cure rates in acute leukemia, testicular cancer, Hodgkin's disease, and lymphatic cancers.

Approximately two decades ago, physicians made a major intellectual breakthrough when they started to perceive that breast cancer was not just a problem confined to the breast itself but rather it was disease that could affect the whole body. (It was systemic.) The concept then developed that to obtain a cure in cancer, it was necessary to destroy each and every cancer cell. A vast amount of clinical research validated the concept that the earlier the diagnosis and the earlier the tumor burden, more specifically, the fewer number of cancer cells, the easier it was to get a high cure rate.

In regard to the role of chemotherapy in breast cancer, there have been literally hundreds of rigorously conducted clinical trials on literally thousands and thousands of women which reveal that the use of chemotherapy can result in increased cure rates ranging from 30-35%. Breast cancer cells are extremely sensitive to the chemotherapeutic drugs. Chemotherapy can be toxic or damaging to all cells, but they are especially effective in destroying cancer cells. The reason is that cancer cells are inherently defective and more sensitive to chemotherapy than normal cells. They are also more easily destroyed because they divide more rapidly than normal cells. One of the great breakthroughs and advances in breast cancer treatment has been the development of over 75 active agents in the treatment of breast cancer. There have also been extensive clinical trials that demonstrate that drugs or chemotherapy are far more effective in combination as opposed to using them as individual agents. Another more simplistic view of this concept is that, if you attack cancer cells with multiple medications that operate by different mechanisms, the cells are far less likely to become resistant or to develop immunity to the chemotherapy; therefore, this leads to increased cure rates in breast cancer. Although the majority of patients with breast cancer present with disease that appears to be limited to the breast, a significant proportion of women eventually develop metastatic breast cancer. Determining one's risk of developing metastatic disease, such as analysis of lymph node status, pathology of the tumor, etc., has already been discussed at length in other chapters. Micrometastatic disease represents the most important remaining challenge in breast cancer therapy. Adjuvant systemic therapy is now considered an integral component of the management of most patients with early stage breast cancer.

The systemic adjuvant therapy is defined as the administration of systemic therapy following definitive local regional treatment (including surgery, radiation therapy, or combination of both to the breast) when there is no evidence of distant tumor spread or metastases, but a high likelihood of disease recurrence. The underlying rationale for the use of systemic therapy as an adjunct to surgery for early stage breast cancer is that patients die despite good local control (surgery and radiation therapy) because blood-borne metastases are present in distant organs prior to the diagnosis. Current knowledge of systemic adjuvant therapy is based on results of over 400 clinical trials which indicate that hormonal therapy and chemotherapy favorably alter the natural history of breast cancer. Optimal treatment for women with early stage breast cancer includes hormonal agents, combination chemotherapy, or both. Determining which patients to treat with adjuvant therapy is based on estimating the risk of recurrence if adjuvant therapy is not given. The thrilling news is that chemotherapy has dramatically increased the cure rates in breast cancer.

SIDE EFFECTS OF CHEMOTHERAPY

Ten to fifteen years ago, chemotherapy was often a terrible experience, but the breakthroughs over the last decade have made chemotherapy a very easy and tolerable experience for the vast majority of cancer patients. The most dreaded complications were Gl toxicity, nausea and vomiting. The main cause of nausea was of massive release of chemicals in the body called histamines, which are stored in the cells lining the gastrointestinal tract. The new antinausea drugs, such as Kytril, Zofran and Anzemet now prevent the release the histamines and largely eliminate vomiting and drastically reduce nausea. I am an avid sailor, and I see far more nausea and vomiting on my sailboat then I ever see in breast cancer patients undergoing chemotherapy. Chemotherapy, of course, can also affect the cells lining the mouth through the rectum. Any sores or infections in these areas are very easily treated, and should be reported to your oncologist immediately.

Of all the side affects of chemotherapy, bone marrow toxicity is the most serious. The bone marrow is the factory for while blood cell, red blood cell, and platelet production. The white blood cells fight infection, the red blood cells carry oxygen to the body, and tissues and the platelets prevent bleeding. Many women being treated with chemotherapy for breast cancer will experience a drop in the white blood cell count between 7 to 14 days after treatment. Therefore, it is vital while on chemotherapy to be alert to the signs of infection, such as fever or shaking chills. You must alert your oncologist immediately if experiencing these symptoms so that he can determine the location of the infection and, more importantly, initiate antibiotic therapy. Infection or fevers are often the first signs of bone marrow suppression.

Another major breakthrough is that we now have medications which are genetically engineered growth factors to stimulate white blood cell production and immunity, such as Neupogen and Leukine, or red blood cell production, such as Epogen, or platelet stimulation with Thrombopoietin. The good news is that these medications can be used to prevent infection (by increasing white blood cell count), anemia or blood cell transfusion (with Epogen), or low platelets and bleeding (with Thrombopoietin).

Understandably, the most distressing symptom for most women undergoing chemotherapy is hair loss (alopecia) or hair thinning. Although frustrating, one positive aspect is that hair loss is always 100% reversible and always temporary. All hair that is lost will completely regrow in a short period of time. The main reason for hair loss is that hair growth from the scalp is largely a matter of protein production and when chemotherapy is given on the day of therapy, it interferes with this production. The destruction of the hair follicle or protein is manifested three to four weeks later after the chemotherapy is given. Once again, the good news is that hair loss is again always temporary.

Other side affects from certain chemotherapeutic agents can be damage to the nerve endings in the feet or hands. This is manifested by numbness and tingling but is slowly reversible. Other side affects can be some mild temporary changes in memory and cognitive skills as well as nonspecific fatigue but again, these are always totally reversible.

Chemotherapy can also cause changes in taste. Patients will particularly have a metallic sensation in their mouth and once again, this symptom is always temporary. If a woman is still menstruating, chemotherapy can cause transient failure of the ovary to produce both estrogen and progesterone, and she may experience a temporary and reversal menopause; however, there are a few women who will go into permanent menopause as a result of chemotherapy. The closer a women is to her own natural menopause, the greater the chance the chemotherapy will precipitate it prematurely.

While receiving chemotherapy, many women want to know if they can continue to work. The answer is determined by many variables, the stress of one's work situation, and the specific chemotherapeutic regimen chosen. All of these are major factors in making this decision. Each individual should determine if she needs to work on a modified schedule or not work at all. Almost all major side effects secondary to chemotherapy occur within the first 24 to 48 hours of treatment. At our center, we often give the chemotherapy on a Friday, and most patients are fully recovered by Monday or Tuesday. After many years' experience, this is a time that one should be caring very carefully for themselves. It is only a brief period of time - three or four months, and it is vital to indulge yourself, go easy, reduce as much stress as possible, consider support groups, and engage friends and loved ones. This is truly a time to pamper yourself.

CHEMOTHERAPEUTIC AGENTS IN TREATING BREAST CANCER

The most common agents in treating breast cancer are cyclophosphamide, methotrexate, 5-fluorouracil, Adriamycin, and the taxanes (Taxol and Taxotere). Overall, combination therapy has been shown to be more effective for adjuvant treatment than single agent chemotherapy. Cytoxan, Methotrexate and 5-FU (CMF) is the most commonly used adjuvant chemotherapy regimen in the world. Also highly effective is the use of Adriamycin, and when combined with Cytoxan (CA) or Cytoxan and 5-FU (CAF), it is even more active than CMF alone. Adriamycin has been found to be especially active in the HER-2/neu positive overexpression patients (the HER-2/neu gene). The use of the taxanes has been especially exciting since it is a very highly active agent in breast cancer. Many clinical trials are now in progress to find the most effective way of using CMF, the anthracyclines, and the taxanes.

This is a wonderfully exciting time in both clinical research and the treatment of breast cancer. There are many breakthroughs we are now offering using our new modern chemotherapeutic methods in breast cancer.

Chapter 21
HORMONES
AND BREAST CANCER

When your teenage sons or daughters act peculiar or bizarre,
And won't clean up their rooms and only eat a chocolate bar,
And when they spend uncounted hours talking on their phones,
It's not the weather, you or dad, it's what is called Hormones.

Now I am not the type to place a blame on just one thing,
But when I see my teenage kids behaving "off the wing",
I soon become convinced that those damn hormones are to blame,
And once they start, I know the kids will never be the same.

Now you may ask, "So what has this to do with getting cancer?"
And I'll reply quite knowingly with this simplistic answer,
"If hormones are so strong that they can make my kids go wild,
Imagine what they'll do to cells when they are multiplied".

The breast cells, like the teenage girls, are going quite berserk.
When they're exposed to hormones, they start to overwork.
And if this happens too darn long, a change may soon occur,
And tumor cells may start to grow, which you cannot deter.

This is the Chapter that many women may turn to first Every week, there's another article about estrogens, tamoxifen, and a whole host of other hormonal compounds written by everyone from experts to inexperts. It's hard to know whom to believe, and frequently even your family physician may not have all the up-to-date information. So it's for this reason I turned to Oncologist, Dr. Bichlien Nguyen, an expert in this area, for her input on the subject. She lectures to patients and to physicians, and in her part of this chapter, gives us a clear understanding of what hormones are, what they do, when you should and shouldn't be taking them.

WHAT ARE HORMONES?

Hormones are any substances that are secreted by glands inside the body. These compounds are then transported to various organs and affect functions of specific susceptible tissues in these organs.

The most important hormones affecting breast tissue are called ESTROGEN and PROGESTERONE.

Every month, a mature egg from an ovary will become mature enough to travel to the uterus and to be fertilized by a sperm. To prepare for this whole process--that is, to get ready for a possible pregnancy--the ovaries produce an enormous amount of estrogen and progesterone. These hormones will then cause tissues lining the uterus to grow, become thickened and filled with blood vessels ready for the embedding of a fertilized egg. They also stimulate breast tissue to grow in anticipation of a pregnancy. If there is no fertilized egg, the ovaries will stop producing estrogen and progesterone. Without the effect of these hormones, especially progesterone, the lining of the uterus will be sloughed off. This is when a woman has her menstrual bleed.

This whole process is what we call a woman's menstrual cycle, which repeats itself from the start of her first menstrual cycle up until menopause. Even after hysterectomy, if they are intact, the ovaries will continue to ovulate, and produce these female hormones in large quantity each month but a woman will not bleed because she has no uterus.

HOW DOES A HORMONE
CAUSE CHANGE IN OTHER ORGANS?

After being produced by the ovaries, estrogen or progesterone will be transported in the blood stream to the breast, the uterus, the bones, the brain, and other organs. The organs are composed of millions of cells, each of which can be compared with a machine that is a part of a huge factory, the organ. Each organ has a different function in the body and may respond differently to the same stimulus.

How are these extremely complicated processes carried out in the body?

It turns out that each of these organs contains tiny different protein structures called receptors. These receptors act like "locks" for these cells, and can be turn on by "keys". These "keys" are the hormones. They fit into their own receptors and "turn on" the machinery of the cells through various complicated signal pathways. Estrogen will only active estrogen receptors and progesterone, its own receptors in breasts.

EFFECTS OF ESTROGEN
AND PROGESTERONE ON THE BREAST

These hormones have tremendous impact on breast tissue. Breast cells have high concentrations of both estrogen and progesterone receptors. During secretory phases of the menstrual cycles or during pregnancy, the enormous amount of estrogen and progesterone will stimulate these receptors, causing swelling of the breasts, increasing blood flow to the breasts, and proliferation of the breast glands. These changes will recede when the hormone effect is gone. When a woman reaches menopause--that is, when her ovaries are no longer active--only a very small amount of female hormones are produced by the adrenal glands (small glands situated right on top of the kidneys) and by fat tissues. The breast glands of menopausal women will become much less dense with less glandular tissue and more fat tissue. If a woman is on hormone replacement therapy, the amount of hormone would be much higher and her breasts may become much denser with more glandular tissues, resembling a younger woman's breasts.

EFFECTS OF ESTROGEN AND PROGESTERONE
ON THE DEVELOPMENT OF BREAST CANCERS

Various studies have indicated that prolonged stimulation of breast tissues by estrogen and progesterone is a strong risk factor in the development of breast cancer. It is thought that by repeated hormone stimulation and growth and division, breast cells will have more opportunity to mutate, that is to become abnormal in their genetic make up, and to become cancerous. The more changes the cells have, the more chance they will become more malignant. For example, with one genetic change a cell may stay normal, but with two changes it will become pre-malignant. More changes in the genetic make-up of the cell may cause frank cancer. A cancer may also transform into a more aggressive type with further genetic changes.

HORMONE-RELATED RISK FACTORS FOR BREAST CANCER

The most common risk factors for breast cancer are hormone-related. These are the following:

Age Most cancers are related to more advanced age because of accumulation of damage to the genes over the years. In case of breast cancer, I believe that the hormone stimulation over the years is also a major factor. If you look at the graph showing age versus breast cancer risk, you can see that the rate increases rapidly while a woman is in her productive years, then start to slow down by the time she reaches menopause when only a small amount of hormone are made. This means that even though we find the most breast cancer in older women, the damage to the cells has been done during her previous years with high hormone stimulation.

Early menarche (having first menstrual cycle at an early age), and *late menopause* are factors related to prolonged exposure to hormone stimulation, and therefore increased in breast cancer risk. The average age at menarche in modern North America is about 12. Several decades ago, it used to be much higher at about age 14 to 15. Better nutrition and faster growth have led to earlier menarche and earlier ovulation. Young girls who are involved in moderate to strenuous physical activities or who have less body fat typically have menarche later at ages 13 or older. They also have less ovulatory cycles than less active girls. Therefore, late menarche is a protective factor from breast cancer. In general, each year that menarche is delayed result in about 20% reduction in risk of breast cancer.

Physical inactivity is an important factor. Adolescents and adults in their productive years who exercise as little as 4 or more hours per week can reduce breast cancer risk (up to the age of 40) by as much as 60%.

Late first pregnancy is believed to be a risk factor while early first pregnancy at 20 years of age or younger has a protective effect. A first trimester abortion, whether induced or spontaneous, increases risk of breast cancer.

Family history of breast cancer is a major risk factor. These women may be genetically predisposed to have higher level of hormones in addition to other genetic factors that influence the development of breast cancer.

Lactation for a long period of time may reduce breast cancer risk.

Weight has a strong relation with breast cancer risk especially in women older than 60. For these women, a 20-pound weight gain will result in an 80% increase in breast cancer risk.

Race is a strong risk factor for breast cancer. Caucasians have higher risk than other races. I believe that it is again related to longer ovulation due to better nutrition as discussed above. For this reason, Japanese women who immigrated to the United States and adopted the new diet would develop risk for breast cancer almost as high as Caucasian women.

Lobular Carcinoma In Situ is a condition that denotes a very high risk to develop breast cancer. Years ago, it was thought to be a non-invasive breast cancer, hence the name "carcinoma in situ". Today, it is no longer considered a cancer or even pre-cancerous, but a marker for high risk of breast cancer development. It is again a marker of hormone stimulation.

Atypical Ductal Hyperplasia is considered a premalignant process. This lesion is composed of breast ducts that have grown under hormone influence and changed into something which is not malignant yet but is not normal either, and may progress with time into cancer if there are more genetic damage in the cell.

Now that we have discussed the effects of hormones on breast cancer risk, let's examine the Risks and Benefits of the most popular hormone treatments for women in the United States, namely Hormone Replacement Therapy and Birth Control Pill.

HORMONE REPLACEMENT THERAPY, YOUR HEALTH, AND RISK OF BREAST CANCER

Hormone replacement therapy (HRT) is the use of exogenous estrogen and progesterone in postmenopausal women who no longer have the capability to produce their own hormones. These hormones are given in different forms: pills, patches on skin or injections. They may be synthetic preparation or made from natural sources such as urine of pregnant mares.

Hormone replacement therapy has been used extensively in the US for the last 20 years with the purpose to protect postmenopausal women from developing coronary heart disease, from osteoporosis (brittle bones), from hot flashes and other changes related to lack of estrogen, however, because of female hormone relationship with the development of breast cancer, there has been many controversial discussion and debate about its routine use for all postmenopausal women. I will go over the possible risks and benefits of Hormone Replacement Therapy.

WHAT ARE THE BENEFITS OF HORMONE REPLACEMENT THERAPY?

Decreased risk of coronary heart disease. Hormone replacement therapy has been shown by many studies to reduce the risk of coronary heart disease by lowering level of the bad cholesterol LDL, and by elevating level of the good cholesterol HDL. However, there are other medications which are much more potent for treating high cholesterol level than hormones. If you have high cholesterol, you should ask your doctor about other alternatives.

Stronger bones. Hormone replacement therapy also keeps the bones stronger and prevents bone fractures which are complications of osteoporosis. Again, if you do have osteoporosis or high risk for osteoporosis such as family history of the disease, or being Caucasian with a slender body frame, Hormone Replacement Therapy may help you. Keep in mind that there are new drugs which are more effective and do not carry risk of breast cancer.

Less menopausal symptoms. When a woman is going through the "change" or menopause, she may experience symptoms caused by a sudden drop of her estrogen and progesterone levels. These symptoms may be hardly noticeable to completely disabling. She may experience hot flush or hot flashes, sweating, depression, irritability, forgetfulness, facial hair growth, dry skin, dry vagina, lower sex drive, urinary symptoms, and so on. Hormone replacement therapy is probably the best available treatment for these symptoms even though it cannot entirely eliminate these symptoms in many cases.

May reduce risk of Alzheimer's disease which is a form of dementia, and mostly a disease of the elderly.

May reduce risk of developing colon cancer, the second most common cancer in women.

May reduce risk of osteoarthritis.

RISKS OF HORMONE REPLACEMENT THERAPY

Breast cancer. This is the most feared side effect of Hormone Replacement Therapy. As we have discussed above, female hormones exert great influence on the breast and the development of breast cancer. However, the 1.7 to 2.5 times higher relative risk of developing breast cancer in women on Hormone Replacement Therapy is considered by many medical experts to be worth taking in order to prevent death from heart disease. On the hand, *many* women have very low risk of developing coronary heart disease or osteoporosis, and may not get any benefit from Hormone Replacement Therapy.

Blood clots. Hormone Replacement Therapy may cause blood clots in blood vessels of the extremities, the brain, and the lungs; causing severe problems such as swelling and painful limbs, respiratory failure, or sometimes strokes. These events are fortunately very rare but do occur, especially in women who are predisposed to develop blood clots. Therefore, it is very important to discuss with your doctor carefully about your medical history, and your family history before starting on Hormone Replacement Therapy.

Uterine cancer. Estrogen by itself promotes growth of the lining of the uterus. Unopposed growth leads to higher risk of developing uterine cancer. Therefore, if a woman is placed on Hormone Replacement Therapy with an intact uterus, her doctor will give her a combination of both estrogen and progesterone. The role of progesterone is to reduce the risk of uterine cancer by promoting the shedding of the uterine lining, and thereby reducing the overgrowth of endometrial cells that could lead to cancer development.

Ovarian cancer. Estrogen by itself may increase the risk of ovarian cancer. Women who have family history of ovarian or breast cancer, or having the breast-ovarian cancer gene BRCA1, or risk factors related to increased ovulation--as described above for breast cancer--- are at higher risk to develop ovarian cancer. These women probably should not use Hormone Replacement Therapy if they have not had their ovaries removed. There is not much data about the effect of progestin on the risk of ovarian cancer at the present time.

Gallstones. Estrogen increases the risk of developing gallstones. If a woman is middle-aged and overweighed, she is at risk for gall- stones, and should be careful in her decision to take Hormone Replacement Therapy. These women may want to use the patch instead of the pill.

Fibroids. These are non-cancerous tumors of the uterus which tend to shrink when a woman's hormone level is low. With Hormone Replacement Therapy, these tumors may grow again and may cause uterine bleeding.

Endometriosis. This is a condition where the cells lining the inside of the uterus somehow escape into the abdomen cavity, outside of the uterus. These tissues may swell under the influence of hormone and cause pain.

Lupus. Hormone therapy may increase the risk of lupus, an autoimmune disease that attacked many different organs.

BIRTH CONTROL PILL AND BREAST CANCER

Birth control pills contain either estrogen or progesterone or both. They may increase the risk of blood clots and gallbladder disease, and they may increase the risk of breast cancer. They are not recommended for women who have history of blood clots including those of the legs, the lung, the brain or the heart. Also, if you smoke, have breast cancer, liver disease or are pregnant, you should not take birth control pills. The advantage of birth control pill is the reduction in the risk of developing ovarian and uterine cancers because the pill suppresses ovulation. And most importantly, it is the best birth control method.

HORMONE MANIPULATION
IN THE TREATMENT OF BREAST CANCER

Breast cancer is usually considered a systemic disease even in fairly early stage when the whole tumor can be resected totally without any microscopically visible residual. The reason is that some cell may have escape the main tumor and spread to other areas of the body, before the main tumor is removed. It is not unusual to see breast cancer coming back many years, sometimes more than 20 years, after surgery of the original tumor. When a cancer has spread beyond the breast, it is usually not feasible to remove the tumor by surgery. A systemic treatment is required. For breast cancer, hormone manipulation has been shown to be very effective in treating the majority of breast cancers, those that express estrogen receptor or progesterone receptor. One of the ways to manipulate the female hormone is to remove its source of production by surgically removing the ovaries. The ovarian function can also be destroyed by radiation therapy or be put on hold temporarily by using injections of a class of drugs called LHRH agonists, of which the most popular are Lupron and Zoladex.

However, the most widely used method of hormone manipulation is a drug called tamoxifen.

Tamoxifen is a synthetic compound that was developed in the early 1960's and since then has been used extensively in the treatment of breast cancer. Tamoxifen has a general structure that resembles the structure of estrogen. It works by binding to the estrogen receptor and preventing the activation of this receptor by estrogen. The drug itself is the "wrong key" (to use the lock and key analogy again) which cannot turn on the machinery of the cell. However, since it fits into and blocks the lock, the right key which is estrogen cannot fit in. Therefore, the cell dies or becomes inactive.

Tamoxifen is quite effective in the treatment of advanced breast cancer. It is also given to women with receptor positive breast cancer that has been totally resected to reduce the chance of its recurrence. For noninvasive breast cancer, tamoxifen can reduce the risk of recurrence by 40%.

Tamoxifen is not the only drug available. Other drugs such as toremifene are also approved to be used in this setting and are equally efficacious in the treatment of breast cancer.

For tumors which have become resistant to tamoxifen, second and third line drugs are available and efficacious. These drugs are Arimidex, letrozole, Megace, and aminoglutethimide. Many more are going through various stages of development and testing and may be found to be even more useful.

TAMOXIFEN AND PREVENTION OF BREAST CANCER

Tamoxifen has an antiestrogenic effect on breast tissue. It has been found recently to reduce the risk of developing breast cancer in high risk women. A national study called Breast Cancer Prevention Trial tested the use of tamoxifen against placebo (dummy pill) in women with high risk for breast using most of the risk factors that I described above. The risk factors used in this trial: Race, age, age of menarche, age of first live birth, the number of first degree relatives with breast cancer, the number of previous breast biopsies, the presence of atypical hyperplasia are entered into a computer model developed by Gail and colleagues to calculated relative risk of developing breast cancer in that particular patient. If a patient is 60 years of age or older; or if she has history of LCIS, she is qualified automatically for this study. This study found that tamoxifen reduces the risk of breast cancer in these women by almost 50% after 4 years of fellow up. A longer follow up time will be necessary to confirm this finding. This model may overestimate the risk Of breast cancer in some women such as those who have a breast biopsy for benign finding while underestimating the risk of women with strong family history. These women may carry one of the genes for breast cancer--BRCAl or BRCA2--that denote very high lifetime risk of breast cancer. However, it is a fairly accurate and quick assessment of a woman's risk. It is also very easy to use in your doctor's office and may provide him or her a handy tool to help in counseling you egarding hormone usage.

OTHER BENEFITS OF TAMOXIFEN

Tamoxifen is antiestrogen in the breast but its effects on the cholesterol levels and the bones are actually similar to estrogen. It means that tamoxifen can protect your heart and bones to some extent.

RISKS OF TAMOXIFEN

The exciting benefit of tamoxifen is dampened by its side effects. Overall, tamoxifen is quite well tolerated. However, it can cause severe hot flashes and other menopausal symptoms described above. In this regard, it is an antiestrogen.

But, it is not quite an antiestrogen in the uterus. Somehow, the effect of tamoxifen on the lining of the uterus is more similar to that of estrogen. It may promote growth of this tissue and can double the risk of uterine cancer. However, you have to put this risk into perspective. If your risk for breast cancer far outweighs the risk of cancer of the uterus, then you may be better off taking tamoxifen.

Uterine cancer can be fatal if it has spread but if you are vigilant and have it detected early, it can be cured by the removal of the uterus (hysterectomy). If you experience any abnormal vaginal bleeding while taking tamoxifen, you should notify your doctor as soon as possible. Your doctor may need to do a pelvic examination and to biopsy the lining of the uterus to see if it has become cancerous or not. Do not panic, however. Keep in mind that most of these bleedings are from benign thickening of the uterus and not from cancer.

WHAT ABOUT RALOXIFENE (EVISTA)?

This is a drug in the same class as tamoxifen with similar side effects except that probably it does not cause uterine cancer. Evista is a drug in the same class as tamoxifen. It has been tested in postmenopausal women with osteoporosis, and was found to reduce the risk of bone fractures in this population. On analysis of the results, it was also found to reduce risk of developing breast cancer in these women by 70% and to have no increase risk of uterine cancer. However, because the drug is new, this side effect may not be obvious in short term follow up and may become more apparent with time. Otherwise, the drug has a similar side-effect profile as tamoxifen, such as hot flashes and blood clots. This drug has not been tested in the treatment of breast cancer and should not be used as a treatment for breast cancer at the present time.

THE QUEST FOR THE PERFECT HORMONE IS STILL GOING

The perfect hormone should be able to control a woman's postmenopausal symptoms; to prevent osteoporosis; to protect the heart; to reduce breast, ovarian, and uterine cancers, and to have very few other side effects. We probably will never be able to produce a perfect hormone but take heart. Across the country, new generations of hormone treatments are tested, and brought to clinical trials regularly. I am optimistic that a near-perfect hormone will be available in a not too far future.

SO, WHAT SHOULD A WOMAN DO ABOUT HORMONE TREATMENT?

See your doctor for a thorough risk assessment and physical examination. A complete medical history--including your own medical history, your symptoms and how they affect you, habits such as smoking or alcohol usage, environmental exposure history, family history of any major illness--is essential in helping your doctor to guide you in the decision to use hormone treatment or not.

A physical examination and laboratory study of your blood and urine may reveal illness that may be unknown to you and help in your treatment plan. After a thorough discussion of risks, a treatment plan can be formulated. This plan should specifically address and be tailored for your individual situation.

Chapter 22
INFUSION CENTER

I visit the Infusion Center today
The service is fine as the Ritz.
I only wish that I could stay
Going home is really the pits!

In the center I'm always treated like royalty
My every need is met,
I think I'll give up my family loyalty
And become the Center's Pet.

They feed me well, there's movies and scones,
I'm spoiled as spoiled can be.
In a way I'll be sad when that final day comes
And I've taken my last therapy.

The Oncology Certified Nurse has studied extensively and received specialized training in working with patients with cancer. It's a highly technical area which encompasses general nursing skills along with psychosocial skills and a broad knowledge of the treatment of cancer, along with its complications and side effects. This individual must recognize every potential problem and must be familiar with all the new oncological drugs on the market today. Frequently the patients are receiving very powerful medications, and the need for expertise and comfortability is at its greatest. Andrea Berman, RN, exemplifies the superbly trained oncology and infusion nurse of today, and gives a fine overview of an Infusion Center in her chapter.

WHAT IS AN INFUSION CENTER?

An Infusion Center is an outpatient facility for providing a patient with any type of intravenous (IV) treatment deemed necessary by a physician. This would include Chemotherapy, IV Hydration, Blood and Blood Products, Antibiotics, and the drawing of blood for laboratory examinations.

And most of all, the staff at the Infusion Center provide a one-on-one personal interaction with patients who are often confused, lonely, apprehensive, and scared. Social workers on the premises provide psychosocial support on an individual basis. A nursing director oversees the operation under the aegis of a physician, and a clinical nurse specialist is available for teaching and referral to other information sources. The patients develop a close relationship with the professional staff in a comfortable setting where they have a private TV, videotapes, and are served meals in a warm atmosphere.

Patients are taught to give their own injections; they are given information about everything from chemotherapy to sexuality issues. The center is affiliated with a hospital for a multiplicity of services and is fully insurance covered. Emergency care is available, if needed. The nurses are Oncology Certified--"they know their stuff"--they know about the drugs used and the possible reactions and side effects, and these nurses can answer the patient's questions about the therapy, and in this way act as an extension of the physician.

During the treatment, a patient's family can stay with her, observing the procedure if desired, and asking any questions.

Now to a more practical problem. Each patient receiving medication may need intravenous medications. Often it is difficult to find good veins in a patient, and so long-term venous access is an area of interest to the patient, nurse, and physician. There are many types of venous access devices, and we will describe some of the more common procedures used for treating cancer patients.

One long-term indwelling catheter is called a PICC line (Peripherally Inserted Central Catheter). It is usually placed with a local anesthetic in the radiology department by a radiologist. Other lines placed by physicians, usually surgeons, in an operating room setting, under local or general anesthesia, are as follows:

The Hickman or Groshong catheter: This is placed through a skin puncture into a vein which leads to a larger central vein. This catheter has an injection port or rubber injection site which is outside the body. Blood samples can be drawn from the catheter, obviating the need for puncturing a vein, and medications and chemotherapy can be given through this site as well. Care must be taken with these catheters to assure patency (that it stays open), and to prevent infection. The catheter needs to be cleansed and dressed regularly, and may need to be flushed with saline or an anticoagulant solution such as heparin. Catheters that become clogged can be unclogged by a physician using special medicines, but if a severe infection occurs, the catheter may have to be removed and replaced.

Another type of intravenous access device is called a Port-A-Cath, which looks like a small button-shaped reservoir under the skin. It is accessed by a special needle called a Gripper which is inserted through the skin into the reservoir. When the needle is removed, because the Port-A-Cath is beneath the skin, no daily cleansing is needed. It does, however, occasionally need to be flushed with saline and heparin to prevent clotting.

Many patients are leery about having these access devices placed. However, once in place, they are very happy with them, and when the treatments are completed, the lines can be removed relatively easily. The Infusion Center nurses are experts in instruction and care of these intravenous access lines, and will notify a physician if any problems arise.

A feeling of community and comraderie develop between the patients in the center, and frequently new patients learn a great deal of personal information from the long-term patients.

The goal of the Infusion Center is to make the patient comfortable, to feel at ease. A frightening situation becomes a safe haven for the patient and family during the necessary treatments. An atmosphere of caring pervades the center.

If patients have to be hospitalized, the medical floor nurse and the oncology nurse work together to make the transfer and transition to inpatient status one with minimal complexity.

Outpatient Infusion Centers are becoming a standard of practice in most major communities, and should be sought after by patients requiring this type of therapy.

The nurses in an Infusion Center are specially trained to handle the complications of the therapy they administer, and perhaps the most unpleasant acute problem is nausea. The following are a few measures recommended at the OCRCC Infusion Center to help patients minimize the extent and severity of chemotherapy-induced nausea and vomiting. The patient will receive medication to prevent nausea, but should she experience even a little nausea, she should tell the nurse or her physician. Keeping the patient free from nausea is the ultimate goal. So these are the recommended measures:

- Eat food served cold or at room temperature.
- Drink clear liquids in severe cases of nausea.
- Sip liquids slowly.
- Eat bland foods.
- Avoid spicy hot foods.
- Rinse mouth with lemon water.
- Avoid sweet, fatty, highly-salted foods.
- Avoid foods with strong odors.
- Avoid eating or drinking 1-2 hours before and after chemotherapy.
- Eat light meals throughout the day.
- Use distractions such as music, television, games, and reading whenever possible.
- Listen to relaxation tapes before, during, and after receiving chemotherapy.
- Employ visual imagery music therapy.
- Sleep during intense periods of nausea.
- Practice good oral hygiene.

The infusion nurses are familiar with your chemotherapy and hormone therapy drugs and their side effects, and can give you literature about each one of them. In addition, they have become experts in the management of pain and nausea along with the pain management specialists and your oncologist, and can discuss different pain medicines with you. The nurses have a large number of drugs available to treat nausea; the common anti-nausea drugs include Decadron, Compazine, Kytril, Zofran, and Reglan.

But not all the treatment is chemotherapy, hormonal, pain and anti-nausea medication. You may be receiving medication to increase the calcium in your bones and prevent osteoporosis (Aredia), drugs which stimulate development of red blood cells (Epogen, Procrit), white blood cells (Neupogen, Leukine), and platelets (Thrombopoetin, Neumega). Prior to chemotherapy, patients are frequently given relaxants such as Ativan, and if any allergic reactions occur to blood or blood products or to another drug, Benadryl is the first drug of choice.

For a somewhat complete list of the most common drugs used in the treatment of cancer, see the Drug list on page 271.

Chapter 23
CANCER RECURRENCE

The cancer, like the cat, came back.
The old tumor train got back on the track.
The damn thing's persistent, but I won't give in,
I'll fight it, despite it, until I can win.

Life is too precious to fall by the way,
So I hold up my head and defiantly say:
"Each day is a blessing which must be revered
And you'll not take it from me, it will not be feared".

In a world of recurrent tumors,
There are too many crazy rumors.

One of the greatest fears of any woman who has been treated in the past for cancer and told that there is no further evidence of active disease, is the fear of recurrence. She has usually pictured in her own mind her physician telling her the bad news in her darkest moments, and regardless of the number of years, that awful seed of doubt has found a small niche somewhere in the back of her brain, and just sets up house there! The size of this "house" and its effect on the woman is often tempered by the actual disease, and by the success or failure of the interaction in a psychosocial program.

And if and when such a recurrence happens, the woman needs not only information but a tremendous support from family, physician, psychosocial services, and most of all--herself.

Some women with recurrent disease are cured, and others with extreme disease are still treatable and have long productive lives. It is important to keep the perspective, recognizing that a productive life is precious, and dying is almost always unpredictable. Dr. Jhangiani, an oncologist who frequently deals with advanced breast cancer in women, is very sensitive to all these issues, and gives us some insight into his therapy in this chapter. But at the outset, let us differentiate between recurrent disease and metastatic disease.

Recurrent disease refers to the recurrence of cancer but it can be local, as in the incisional area or chest wall, or it can be a distant spread such as in the bones or liver, which we call metastatic disease.

Local recurrence may be from residual tumor cells that remained from the original surgery and grew over subsequent months or years or local recurrent growth in surrounding skin edges. These types of tumor growth can often be treated by surgical resection along with radiation and chemotherapy, and may result in complete eradication of the cancer and cure of the disease.

But when we talk about metastatic breast cancer, we are discussing an entirely different matter. This is breast cancer which has gone beyond local control and spread beyond our ability to give the patient a complete cure, although with appropriate treatment, the life expectancy of many of these women can be many years.

So let us progress to some information by oncologist, Dr. Haresh Jhangiani, who is faced with this difficult problem on a daily basis.

BREAST CANCER RECURRENCE AND METASTATIC DISEASE

Metastatic breast disease remains a major challenge and it continues to be a significant and growing problem in the world. Despite modern and technological improvements, over half the population diagnosed with breast cancer will, at some stage, have a recurrence of their breast cancer.

Although there is no curative treatment for metastatic breast disease, effective measures to provide meaningful palliation and elongation of life do exist. A combination of radiation therapy, chemotherapy, newer drug combinations, and improved biological therapeutics have significantly improved the quality of life.

NATURAL HISTORY

Breast cancer is most likely to recur in liver, lungs, and bones. The site of relapse is often close to the original tumor, but this location may depend on the interval between the initial diagnosis and recurrence of disease. Patients who are cancer-free for over two years often have bony metastases, and patients who are cancer-free for one year or less often present with liver and lung metastases. Adjuvant chemotherapy (therapy given to patients when first diagnosed with breast cancer) has positively impacted the pattern of relapse. Although metastatic breast disease is incurable, patients who present with liver and lung metastases may not do as well as those with bony disease. The site of disease is associated with survival. There is a wide variation in survival times within the subsets of patient populations, and can range from one to twenty-four months with patients who present with liver or lung metastases and survival time can range from six months to eight years in patients who have only bony disease. Breast cancer is a very hydrogenous disease, and the prognosis of patients frequently varies significantly.

DIAGNOSTIC WORK-UP

Patients newly diagnosed with breast cancer should have the following tests done at recurrence: A chest x-ray, bone scan, CAT scan of the abdomen, a complete blood count including chemistry panel, liver function tests, calcium, CEA, tumor markers, CA-127, and a complete physical examination. Other testing is indicated depending on the patient's history and other manifestations. It is essential that biopsies be done to confirm the recurrence. At times, benign disease can be mistaken for metastatic disease and other secondary forms of tumors may be diagnosed. Tumors can also undergo biological transformation and, therefore, the first site of metastatic disease should be biopsied. The site most accessible should be biopsied in the least invasive manner. Tumor markers essentially aid the clinician in monitoring the response to therapy. These tumor markers are not diagnostic tests, and should not be used as tools to diagnose recurrences.

THE TREATMENT

Metastatic breast disease is incurable. The goal of therapy is, therefore, effective palliation with the least degree of toxicity. The various therapies include hormonal therapies, chemotherapies, and biologicals. Radiation therapy also plays a role in patients who present with metastatic disease, and this will be discussed by other authors in the book.

HORMONAL THERAPY

Antihormonal therapy for breast cancer was first described in 1896 by Dr. Beata, who then treated a woman with metastatic breast disease by removal of ovaries, and demonstrated that these tumor nodules on the skin regressed. Since then, various surgical approaches have been used to cause hormonal blocking. With the advent of oral hormonal agents, surgical castration is no longer employed routinely in patients with metastatic breast disease. The expression of estrogen/progesterone antigen (protein) correlates with effectiveness of hormonal agents. The response rate varies from 10-70%, and the duration of response is approximately 16-18 months. Patients who express estrogen/progesterone proteins on the cancer cells have the best prognosis. Ten percent of patients who do not express this protein will also respond to hormonal manipulation.

HORMONAL AGENT – TAMOXIFEN

Tamoxifen is a synthetic antiestrogen that binds the estrogen receptor. It is safe and effective, and the response rate varies from 16-52%, depending on the estrogen/progesterone positivity. A daily dose of 20 mg is sufficient enough; most patients are prescribed 10 mg twice daily. Although tamoxifen is an antiestrogen, it also has estrogen-like activity that accounts for secondary benefits. Other potential benefits include the preservation of bone density, reduction of cholesterol levels with a decrease in the cardiovascular morbidity, and decrease in secondary primary breast tumors. The side effects of the medication include increase in hot flashes, increased vaginal secretions, less than 20% incidence of thromboembolic events, although this side effect needs to be evaluated closely because patients with metastatic breast disease are at increased risk for thrombotic event. The risk of endometrial carcinoma needs to be evaluated closely in patients with metastatic breast disease as they are also at an increased risk for uterine cancer. There is some animal data suggesting that tamoxifen can also cause liver cancer but the incidence in humans has not been reported. There have also been some reports of retinal and corneal changes with tamoxifen.

PROGESTERONAL AGENTS

Progesterone has also been shown to induce response in metastatic breast disease. The commonly used drug is Megace which interferes with binding to estrogen receptors. It also accelerates the destruction of estrogen, and interferes with conversion of other Androgens to estrogens. The response rate with Megace is 25-40% in free-treated patients. The response rate for most hormonal agents are very similar in patients who are given these drugs as first line; however, the response rate decreases significantly when they are used as second and third line agents. Also, the response duration continues to diminish when used as second and third line agents. The side effects of progesterone include weight gain, vaginal bleeding, fluid retention, thromboembolic phenomena. Weight gain is the most distressing side effect of progesterone. It is as effective as tamoxifen as first line but is rather inconvenient as it is administered four times daily, although single daily doses can be administered.

AROMATASE INHIBITORS

What are the hormones that kill cancer cells by blocking estrogen? Aminoglutethimide is an effective agent for the treatment of breast cancer but is not a pure aromatase inhibitor, and does frequently require concomitant administration of steroids. In the last several years, other aromatase inhibitors have been used, and these include Formestane which is sixty times more potent than aminoglutethimide. This drug inhibits the circulating estrogen levels in postmenopausal women by 60%, but has little effect on the suppression of estrogen in premenopausal women. The oral response rate in phase II trials was in the range of 7-40%. The most common side effects are again hot flashes, lethargy, rash, and dizziness.

Other hormonal agents used are androgens and sometimes luteinizing hormone agonists to suppress the ovarian production of estradiol or desensitizing the receptors. Patients who benefit the most from hormonal treatments are patients whose tumors express the estrogen and progesterone receptor proteins on tumor cells. Hormone treatment is often used in patients who have noncritical disease, such as bony soft tissue metastases. Patients who are postmenopausal can benefit the best with hormonal manipulations. Occasionally, patients who do not express estrogen and progesterone receptor proteins are treated with androgenous hormones, and these patients have a very low response rate in the range of 10%.

CHEMOTHERAPY

Many agents are available in the treatment of metastatic breast disease. Adriamycin, is the oldest and most widely used anthracycline. As a single agent, the response rate varies from 40-50% in treated patients. This response rate can be increased when it is used in combination with other agents such as Cytoxan, Methotrexate, Taxol or Taxotere. Cytoxan and Adriamycin are the most commonly used combination, followed by Adriamycin in combination with Taxol or Taxotere. Over the years, many other anthracyclines have been used, which include mitoxantrone, epirubicin, and idarubicin.

And so we conclude Dr. Jhangiani's section. The didactic treatment of metastatic disease is well documented in many texts, journals, and on the Internet. But a comprehensive approach to the management of this most serious of breast cancer conditions is what I want to stress in the conclusion to this chapter. It is not just cancer treatment but the quality of life with which we are concerned. Treatment must be accompanied by a clear awareness of patient comfort, and close interaction with a support group, a caring physician and our loved ones. I speak from personal family experience when I relate the story of a woman who developed a certain kind of cancer which had spread beyond the limits of curability from the outset of her diagnosis. She was a psychotherapist herself, and yet she was unable to seek out any guidance or help, and the cancer program which treated her did not offer that service. From the time of her diagnosis, she dressed in black, became severely depressed, and essentially exited from the world of the living, isolating herself from friends and relations. She appeared to be waiting each day for her death, and gave up living for the three years that she survived after her diagnosis. This may seem an extreme case, but it happened in my own family to a cousin who, until her disease "struck", loved life, and lived happily with a husband and child. What we need to stress is that our lives are truly a gift, given one day at a time, and much like the adage from that famed support group, AA (Alcoholics Anonymous), we really only have today, and should make the very best of it.

I frequently refer to an ancient poem, from the Sanskrit, which I first read in the book "A Way Of Life" by the famous physician, Dr. William Osler:

The Salutation of the Dawn

Listen to the Exhortation of the Dawn!
Look to this day!
For it is Life, the very Life if Life.
In its brief Course lie all the
Varieties and Realities of your Existence:
The Bliss of Growth,
The Glory of Action,
The Splendour of Beauty;
For Yesterday is but a Dream,
And Tomorrow is only a Vision,
But Today well lived makes
Every Yesterday a Dream of Happiness,
And every Tomorrow a Vision of Hope.
Look well, therefore, to this Day.
Such is the Salutation of the Dawn.

Chapter 24
RESEARCH

Who needs research, anyway?
Black's black, white's white, so who needs gray?
What was good enough for dad, is good enough for me,
Without all this nonsense you call chemistry.

I can't understand why you have all this stuff
I'm not easy to fool or easy to bluff.
I'm a firm believer in my father's firm warning:
"Take two aspirins, then come and see me in the morning!"

S o what's the big deal about research? You say you have cancer; so why bother with this?

Good question!

Actually, the most foresighted Cancer Centers and the most up-to-date oncologists have research as their "middle name". They know that progress is made in the treatment of cancer on a regular basis, and to be at the cutting edge of the treatment spectrum, they need to be aware of what is new, and to be ready to have certain of their patients participate in what we call research protocols or clinical trials.

The pharmaceutical Companies and Medical Centers are involved in basic research science experiments to determine new information about the growth and development of cancer cells. This experimentation, often done first on laboratory animals and in tissue cultures, is frequently the basis for understanding more about the cells, and thereby how to develop drugs and treatments which will destroy these cells. A drug's action may be against a specific cell function such as multiplication or nutrition of a cell, and a specific drug may act to interfere with the ability of a cell to reproduce and eventually cause its death. Recent studies have shown that some drugs prevent angiogenesis, or the ability of a tumor to develop a blood supply to itself; without adequate blood supply, a tumor may die.

So basic research sets the basis for eventual clinical research, and millions of dollars are spent trying out thousands of compounds before a successful one is found. When such a substance is found, it has to be evaluated for its effects, its side effects, and the constancy of its action before it can be proposed for use in humans. And which patients will have these trial drugs? Let us examine this closely.

In early cancers and cancers which are readily curable with the standard surgery, radiation or drug regimens, there is usually no place for the experimental drug. But in a woman with advanced disease, where the physician is losing ground with the usual and standard regimens, there may be a role for carefully conducted and controlled clinical trials called clinical experimentation.

We will discuss now what is called the Three Phases of Clinical Investigative Drug Trials for humans. *Phase I* trials or tests are when a certain promising drug or procedure is tested in a human to determine if it is safe to use, and what are the effective dosages and tolerances. Basically, is the drug or procedure safe to use in humans? Now remember, chemotherapeutic agents are "strong medicines", and will have some unpleasant side effects; the researcher must evaluate the safety along with the side effects and the efficacy. If the drug or treatment has been determined to be safe through clinical trials, then it is brought to *Phase II* trial which measures the objective response rate to the substance or procedure, which in the case of a drug is determined by a significant decrease in the size of the tumor, or in some cases a decrease in the symptoms. Because of the experimental nature of this treatment, it is usually reserved only for patients with advanced cancer.

If the drug or procedure passes Phases I and II, it is ready for a *Phase III* trial. In this study, the new agent or procedure is tested against a standard treatment drug or procedure to compare its effectiveness. These trials may be used in some women with newly diagnosed breast cancer.

Now I should emphasize that these trials are not used just for anti-cancer drugs but also for medications against nausea, pain, and side effects encountered by patients undergoing chemotherapy or symptoms secondary to their tumors. New anti-nausea medications and analgesics are developed in this way for new usage.

If you have breast cancer, you want the best treatment available, and the advances in treatment come from these types of clinical trials. Remember, these studies should only be done by physicians affiliated with major groups such as the NSABP, NCI or SWOG, and University or Major Cancer Centers where the studies are closely monitored and done in a non-biased, scientifically verifiable manner.

Treatment with drugs should no longer be on the basis of one doctor's "I think this is best" philosophy but on the collective conclusions drawn from thousands of patients and many physicians in clinical trials. Women who have participated in clinical trials over the past fifty years have helped themselves as well as the women who come after them Look at the wonderful advances that have been made in the treatment of breast cancer as a result of the work of Dr. Bernard Fisher in the NSABP. He and his colleagues showed that the breast preserving surgeries of lumpectomy and axillary dissection along with postoperative radiation therapy have the same success rate as the old modified and radical mastectomies, and therefore, we are now able to do lesser procedures with better cosmetic and psychosocial results. The newer drugs, such as Taxol and the breast cancer prevention studies with Tamoxifen, have come out of clinical trials!

So, is research a big deal? You bet. It is probably the most important aspect of cancer treatment ever So don't shy away from clinical trials if you think you might be a candidate. Discuss the pros and cons with your oncologist, read the protocol, and make an informed decision.

Chapter 25
RADIATION THERAPY

Radiation...that's the word,
For something neither seen nor heard.
And all the little cancer cells
Don't know what sent 'em down to Hell.

When I was in college, I had to take a course in physics in order to get into medical school. Having been an English and American Literature Major, I left this class to my senior year, and had already been accepted into medical school when I started to take the course. My acceptance to medical school was contingent upon my doing well in my remaining classes as a college senior, and I managed to do well in everything except Physics. I enjoyed the subject matter immensely but when it came to inclined planes and angular momentum and other such "Greek" nonsense, I just couldn't cut the mustard. Physics is an exacting science but my answers were always just a little bit off.

My professor knew about my predicament and eventually I passed satisfactorily with a comment from him that I'd probably make a good doctor, but he knew for sure I'd make a lousy physicist...he wished me well, and I thank him to this day. Anyway – what's all this got to do with Radiation Therapy?

Radiation Therapy is basically a practical application of physics to the practice of medicine, and definitely not the field for me. Radiation Oncologists are the physicians who utilize the high energy generated by special machines, to produce rays which can kill cancer cells. The early treatments by radiation therapy occurred accidentally on purpose in Hiroshima and Nagasaki when all the side effects of radiation were recorded. What the Radiation Oncologists give the patient today is a controlled, accurately directed dosage of radiation which requires a high degree of understanding of physics as well as knowledge of medicine and radiology.

I recall envying those college classmates who found physics simple, and today I find myself envying the skills of radiation oncologist, Dr. Robert Woodhouse, a compassionate, brilliant physician whom I am sure did well at inclined planes and angular momentum. He frequently lectures to patients and physicians as well as discussing his treatments at the Breast Cancer Tumor board along with this associate, Dr. Donald Karon.

Here is Dr. Woodhouse's chapter on Radiation Therapy, and may the force be with you.

RADIATION THERAPY IN BREAST CANCER

For oncologists, the study of breast cancer has been, and continues to be, one of the most challenging projects in cancer medicine. On the one hand, breast malignancy is very prevalent in our society, occurring in about one of eight women nationwide over a lifetime. It remains the most common malignancy in women, with nearly 180,000 new cases in 1998, and the second most lethal malignancy for women, with nearly 44,000 deaths in 1998. On the other hand, arguably we have made more progress in the last 10 years in early diagnosis, treatment, and basic research including genetics of this disease than any other malignancy, and we are now seeing suggestions of improved survival as a result. One of those advances--the use of radiation therapy in early breast cancer--allows more women to avoid mastectomy and preserve their breasts, or prevent the return of disease on the chest wall after mastectomy for advanced cancer.

We are all bombarded by radiation every day—cosmic radiation from the universe, low energy x-rays from TV and computer screens, microwaves from power lines, radio waves from cell phones, and even natural radiation from radium and other trace elements in the soil in some parts of the country. Only in the past 100 years have we learned to "control" radiation and use it, regrettably sometimes destructively, but more often constructively to treat malignant disease.

X-rays were discovered in 1895 by Conrad Roentgen and natural radium was identified in 1898. These newly discovered forms of energy were quickly shown to have effects on human tissue, often by accident, such as the researcher who carried a radium source in his pocket for several hours, and then developed redness and ulceration of the skin. In the early 1900's, this kind of research was channeled into cancer treatment, as rapidly dividing cancer cells were found to respond to radiation.

Breast cancer in the early 1900's was usually a lethal disease. Without the ability to diagnose it early, tumors were advanced and often metastatic at diagnosis, and, in the absence of effective other treatments, rarely controllable with surgery. Utilizing primitive X-ray tubes, however, locally advanced tumors could be shrunk with radiation, though not controlled, and surgery remained the only form of effective therapy through most of the 20th Century. In the last years of this century, research and technology have changed our ways of approaching this disease. Improved diagnostic imaging has allowed identification of early, small cancers, and multiple large studies have confirmed that the results with radiation and mastectomy are equivalent. We can now offer radiation with breast preservation, allowing women to avoid total mastectomy, yet enjoy a high likelihood of life-long control (it is still hard for an oncologist to say "cure" for this disease!).

WHO IS A CANDIDATE FOR RADIATION THERAPY FOR BREAST CANCER?

Most women who are found to have a tumor less than 2 centimeters (cm) in size, the diameter of a nickel, or even larger, and are medically able to undergo removal of the tumor from her breast (lumpectomy) usually in conjunction with removal of some or all lymph nodes in the axilla, is a candidate. Radiation can control 90% or more of these tumors, and prevent their recurrence in the breast, probably for the lifetime of the patient. For the best results, the entire tumor must be removed with clear margins all around.

Not all patients are good candidates for this "breast conservation" procedure; patients with very small breasts may require a near-mastectomy to clear the tumor, losing the cosmetic effect of breast preservation. Patients with very large breasts which drape down the chest are difficult to treat with radiation without higher risks of side-effects including scarring and retraction of the treated breast which may feel hard rather than soft to the touch. Such patients are best treated with mastectomy. Other absolute contraindications include pregnancy at the time of diagnosis, or prior radiation to the thorax, as for Hodgkin's Disease or lung cancer.

"Relative" contraindications, which do not ABSOLUTELY rule out breast conservation, include diffuse disease in a large area of the breast, inability to totally clear margins around the tumor surgically, and collagen vascular disease such as scleroderma or lupus.

WHAT IS THE RADIATION EQUIPMENT LIKE?

Most radiation treatments are given with large machines called "linear accelerators". They are able to produce beams of radiation 100 times more energetic than diagnostic X-rays. These "photon" beams penetrate deeply through tissue but disappear like a beam of light in the sky, so the patient is never 'radioactive'. The beam interacts with all tissue in the path, damaging both normal and cancerous cells. The normal cells are better able to repair the damage, and by treating daily over a period of weeks, the damage builds up in cancer cells, which die when they try to replicate.

In some places a special form of radiation called an "electron" beam is used. Instead of photons which are like X-rays, electrons are actually particles which are accelerated nearly to the speed of light. Instead of passing through tissue like a light beam passes through the air, the electrons are absorbed in a few centimeters of tissue. If breast tumors are near the surface, electron beams can deliver a high dose of radiation to the tumor without penetrating to the lung or heart.

Radioactive implants were popular 10-15 years ago, and are still sometimes used to "boost" the dose of radiation to the tumor. In this case a linear accelerator gives external radiation for about 5 weeks. Then the patient is hospitalized and under anesthesia, plastic tubes containing radioactive sources are placed through the skin into the tumor cavity (the lumpectomy has removed the tumor itself) and left in place for 48-60 hours. These radioactive sources deliver a steady dose of radiation which penetrates only a short distance and again spares vital organs. All techniques give the same overall results and the risks are limited.

HOW DOES THE RADIATION PROCESS BEGIN?

When possible the radiation oncologist would like to see the patient before surgery to assess the disease and discuss the side effects, as well as assure the ability to treat the patient effectively. The patient will usually be referred for treatment 10-14 days after surgery, or when the surgeon feels the incision is healed. If chemotherapy is to be given, the referral may be delayed until chemotherapy is partially or fully completed, from 3-8 months after surgery. The initial consultation is to introduce the patient to the doctor, obtain history and physical exam, and discuss the potential side effects and treatment plan.

On the first treatment day, the patient undergoes a "simulation" or practice set-up to make sure all critical areas are covered by the radiation field, with the least possible treatment of normal vital organs, especially the lung and heart which are near the breast.

X-rays are taken and when approved small pinpoint tattoos are placed on the chest to localize the exact borders of the treatment field for precise reproducibility on a daily basis. This process takes about 1 hour. All other treatments take only a few minutes, and the total time daily in and out of the department is about 20-30 minutes. The total number of treatments depends on the size and aggressiveness of the tumor—smaller tumors take about 7 weeks, and larger tumors take almost 8 weeks for optimal results. This "fractionation" of the radiation treatments is necessary to allow normal tissues inside the radiation field to heal any radiation damage between treatments. Treatments are given only weekdays routinely, with the weekends allowing further healing of normal tissue effects.

WHAT ARE THE POSSIBLE SIDE EFFECTS?

The only side effect everybody experiences is the time commitment; treatments usually take 6 ½ to 8 weeks, 5 days a week, Monday through Friday. While this time commitment is unfortunate, most patients can drive back and forth, and live their lives normally the rest of the day. Treatments can even usually be tailored around jobs, so patients have as little disruption of their lives as possible.

Other side effects most patients experience include tanning or burning of the skin within the treatment field, similar to the sun's effects. This reaction usually begins 3-4 weeks into treatment, and begins to resolve a week or two after completion. The skin reaction is seen first often as a "bumpy" redness in the upper inner portion of the treated breast, which then becomes a well-defined rectangle surrounding the breast. The most intensely involved areas are the inframammary crease and the axilla--where skin surfaces rub against each other, where sweat may accumulate, and where air circulation is poor. A water-based gel such as Aquaphor can help moisturize the skin, but other medications including aloe vera, the plant or gel preparation, or vitamin E are also useful, as are Desitin, or other baby cream. Cortisone is useful for itching, as is Benadryl. Occasionally the skin will peel, and less often a moist breakdown, like blistering after a bad sunburn, occurs usually in patients also receiving chemotherapy. Patients who receive chemotherapy either before or concurrent with radiation may have more severe radiation reactions which may require a short treatment break, a few days to no more than a week usually. These short breaks allow reactions to resolve, and do not reduce the chance for controlling the tumor. Cornstarch helps dry and soothe the affected area until it heals in a week or so. After healing, the area rarely breaks down a second time.

Effects in lung tissue can be potentially serious, especially for smokers, or patients with other lung disease such as asthma or emphysema with reduced lung function. The lung lies beneath the breast, and though the radiation fields are aimed diagonally across the chest, it is impossible to avoid scatter of some radiation into the lung. Symptoms occur in a very small percentage of patients, and may be limited to a short period of dry cough or shortness of breath, like a cold, which disappear spontaneously after 7-10 days.

Some patients may experience a sore throat 4-5 weeks into treatment, usually smokers, or significant alcohol consumers, due to scatter of the radiation beam into the upper esophagus or trachea. These symptoms are usually mild and respond to mild analgesics, or liquid Xylocaine.

Many patients describe a "fatigue" or lack of energy which comes on later in the radiation course, but energy essentially always returns after treatment is completed. Patients may develop a slight drop in blood counts, especially white blood cells and platelets. These counts do not drop as much as with chemotherapy, but may add to the effects of chemotherapy on the blood.

WHAT ABOUT LONG-TERM RISKS?

Radiation therapy is not totally risk-free. A small percentage of patients may experience long-term effects with chronic symptoms. Some sensitive patients will develop a pneumonia-like syndrome with dry cough or shortness of breath which usually resolves within 7-10 days, but on occasion it may persist and require antibiotics and/or steroids, and may cause permanent changes on a chest X-ray. Some patients may develop swelling or redness of the treated breast which usually resolves, but may require antibiotics and may occasionally become permanent.

Lymphedema, or swelling due to lymphatic accumulation, occurs occasionally in the arm after mastectomy, or when an extensive lymph node dissection is performed, especially if there are significant cancer deposits in the lymph nodes. The risk increases if radiation is used to treat the lymph node drainage in the neck. Lymphedema can be a very distressing symptom, but may be at least partially alleviated by an active physical therapy program, diuretics, and compression techniques for the affected arm.

Radiation fields are aimed diagonally across the chest to avoid the lung and heart. However when the left breast is treated, the heart may beat in and out of the field. Some reports suggest an increased risk of coronary artery disease in patients many years after radiation, but it is hard to determine whether the radiation itself was the cause rather than diet, lifestyle or other causes of heart disease. Some reports have also suggested a risk of rib fractures near the treated breast. It is possible that rarely radiation could locally damage the blood supply to a rib, making it weaker and more susceptible to damage with trauma. While these consequences are serious, they happen rarely. The vast majority of patients are able to benefit from breast preservation without serious consequences.

CAN RADIATION BE USED IN OTHER CIRCUMSTANCES?

So far we have only discussed radiation after "lumpectomy" for smaller cancers of the breast. In at least two other circumstances radiation can be used with surgery and/or chemotherapy to help patients with larger tumors.

If a patient undergoes mastectomy and is found to have multiple lymph nodes with cancer in the axilla, or has a breast tumor 4-5 cm. or larger, or the tumor is "high-grade" (meaning it appears more aggressive), there is a very high risk of recurrence of the tumor on the chest wall or in the mastectomy scar, perhaps as high as 40-50%, despite excellent surgery. In the 1960's and 1970's, radiation was used commonly after mastectomy to reduce this risk. In the 1980's, however, its popularity diminished because multiple studies suggested that while radiation was effective in markedly reducing cancer in the chest wall, it did not appear to help patients live longer with advanced disease, and the medical oncologists felt that radiation made it difficult to give full doses of chemotherapy. In the past two years, two studies have now suggested that radiation *does* help patients live longer as well as preventing cancer from recurring on the chest wall. As a result, patients are once again often advised to undergo radiation to the chest wall if multiple nodes are found, if residual cancer is left behind at mastectomy, if the tumor is high-grade, or if other pathological features suggest a high risk of local recurrence.

On occasion, patients present with tumors so large or with "inflammatory" features suggesting infiltration of tumor cells into the lymphatic channels of the skin itself, that surgery is not felt to be the best first treatment; combinations of chemotherapy, often coupled with radiation, may make the tumors markedly shrink, or even disappear, either making surgery possible or avoiding it altogether in some patients.

The past 10 years have brought remarkable changes in the standard treatment of breast cancer, and we are now beginning to see more tumors diagnosed earlier, when the chance for "cure" is the greatest. We anticipate that the early 21st Century will show even more progress in dealing with this disease.

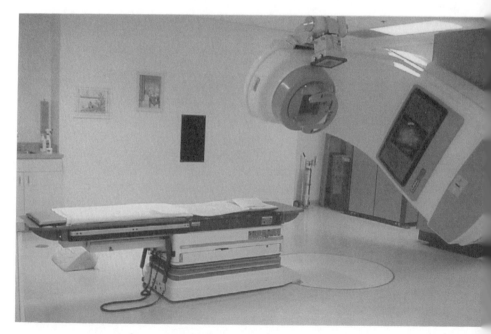

Figure 51. RADIATION THERAPY MACHINE.

Chapter 26
STEM CELL
TRANSPLANTATION

Stem Cells they're called, or Bone Marrow cells
The water of life from your own body's wells
They're vital for making some products one needs
You can think of them now as the blood making seeds.

So we can collect 'em and store 'em in vials
Then give you your therapy in giant piles
And then when you're sick and flat on your back,
We'll thaw 'em and give 'em right back in one crack.

And we have found out, and you soon will discover
This regimen helps you to quickly recover.
So the next time you hear about a stem cell rescue
You'll know they're not talking about a dog named Stem Cell
(Bless you!)

S tem Cell Transplantation is a way of talking about high dose chemotherapy. You may even have heard about Bone Marrow Transplantation--pretty much the same thing, as I will show you. When clinicians found that they could give chemotherapeutic drugs to destroy cancer cells, some scientists felt that if a little was good, maybe a lot is better. The basic principle was a good one; more cancer cells were destroyed in experimental animals with higher doses of certain drugs. The bad part was that the powerful drugs often caused severe damage or even total destruction of the bone marrow. The bone marrow, you may recall, contains the cells that produce blood cells. Under normal circumstances these cells are produced, enter the blood stream, perform for several weeks, and then are destroyed by the healthy human body. Therefore, if the high doses of chemotherapy are to be used, something must be done to prevent the total destruction of the bone marrow cells. Researchers found that if they took some of these "stem cells" or "bone marrow" cells from a patient before giving the high dose chemotherapy, and then reinfusing them after the treatment was completed, they would be rescuing the bone marrow from destruction. This type of treatment has been used in many types of cancer as well as breast cancer, and was initially only used in patients with extensive and metastatic malignancies. Early in this therapy, oncologists would actually remove cells from the bone marrow for storage, but now methods have been devised which allows us to get the stem cells from the peripheral blood (i.e., by removing blood from a vein) in a much less difficult and less painful procedure.

After several clinical trials, stem cell transplantation became recommended for women with high risk breast cancers who had more than 10 (cancer) involved axillary lymph nodes, and in patients who had large cancers (greater than 5 centimeters in diameter). The early data was very supportive for the use of this procedure with prolonged remissions, but longer follow-up has been somewhat disappointing in that most of the women were not totally cured of their cancer. So recent articles in medical journals and lay magazines have put a temporary hold on the use of stem cell transplantation and high dose chemotherapy for breast cancer until further studies can be done. Remember, this type of treatment is very toxic because it is so aggressive and unless the advantages can be clearly demonstrated, its use must be very limited and carefully evaluated by a Tumor Board.

We should also emphasize that this type of treatment can only be performed by specially trained oncologists at centers of excellence which have been established for this purpose. Dr. Jhangiani, who performs this procedure on patients with many types of cancers at our institution, spent many months in training, and has developed a careful protocol for all the patients, and provided special training for the nurses as well as establishing routines in the Infusion Center and in the hospital. While much of the treatment can be done as an outpatient, the patients have to be monitored very carefully for signs of excess toxicity and infection, which means immediate hospitalization and vigorous treatment of the problems.

You should also know that this is a very expensive procedure, and while many insurance companies are covering the procedure for other cancers, several have stopped coverage for breast cancer because of the recent disappointing results. As you know, new and exciting advances are being made in this field, and in the months and years to come the use of high dose chemotherapy and stem cell transplantation may be entirely eliminated or established as an important, effective and safe modality.

Chapter 27
THE AMERICAN
CANCER SOCIETY

Do you want to be a society girl?
Learn how to knit and learn how to purl?
Become a favorite of Emily Post?
Know how to flaunt and know how to boast?

Do you want to drink tea from an old Limoge cup?
Will you only have friends that you know married Up?
And when you have soirees and host fashion balls
Will you always be ready when society calls?

Cause if you want answers to all of the above,
Don't think that you'll find it for money or love,
At the ACS Center for all information,
Where volunteers come from all over the nation.

For this is a society with no false pretenses,
It's only for people who've come to their senses,
And want to give service to help those in need,
It takes a "society girl" of a new special breed.

So if you're concerned more with helping than manners
And don't wave your diamonds, but wave self help banners
Then come to your local ACS Info Center
You'll feel a lot better and much more contenter!

THE ROLE OF THE AMERICAN CANCER SOCIETY
INFORMATION CENTER IN A CANCER CENTER

Basically, when you come down to it, there are three things we're interested in: Diagnosis, treatment, and information. One of the central roles of the American Cancer Society is information; and not just any information but valid information that you can rely upon while floundering in a sea of misinformation and exaggeration. In addition to the multiple services you will learn about in this chapter, I must emphasize that you will be steered in the direction of accurate source material, much of it published by the American Cancer Society itself, as well as books, tapes, and Internet accessibility. This is, to a large degree, a volunteer organization of men and women who get a great satisfaction carrying on a tradition of selflessness and helping. Joanne O'Heany has been instrumental in setting up the vast Information Center at our Medical Center and has been able to, through her own efforts, expand a pilot program into one which is exemplary throughout the nation.

She participates in the Comprehensive Program and has been active in bringing many individuals into the sphere of volunteer participation. Her input in this chapter is exemplary of her work in the Information Center, on Hospital Committees, and in Numerous Cancer Support Groups.

The lives of cancer patients and their families are significantly disrupted by a cancer diagnosis. Long-term treatment creates hardships and difficulties for patients including emotional, physical, and financial problems. The medical community focuses on treatment, and as a result, patients may be uncertain where to turn for help with many of these related problems. Patients treated in distant cancer centers, as well as those treated nearby, may not know where to turn for help in their communities. Resources, information, and guidance offered by this program can be a great benefit for families in crisis. The volunteers are knowledgeable helpers and sympathetic listeners.

Quality information gives people a greater sense of control over their lives at a time when their lives seem out of control. Access to literature and educational programs that reveal cancer facts, treatments, and rehabilitation programs may dispel many common myths, and can relieve patients and families of many unwarranted and realistic fears.

Volunteers direct patients and families to services and resources. These might include early cancer detection programs, support groups, smoking cessation classes, home care, and patient transportation.

Recent changes in cancer treatment and health care delivery have prompted greater demands for the American Cancer Society Information Center's services.

Treatment advances have resulted in increased cure rates and more cancer survivor requiring information, services, support, and rehabilitation. Also, shorter hospital stays for many cancer patients create greater needs for home care, information, and service referrals to ease the transition from hospital to home and to insure the continuity of care.

REACH TO RECOVERY

This is a program of the American Cancer Society which helps women with breast cancer cope with their diagnosis, treatment, and recovery.

The ever-changing medical environment has added new concerns for patients regarding treatment options, informed consent, shorter hospital stays, and insurance coverage.

The newly diagnosed breast cancer patient may feel overwhelmed, vulnerable and alone. A woman needs to feel confident that the treatment she has chosen is the correct one for her.

A visit from a Reach to Recovery volunteer helps a breast cancer patient meet the emotional, physical, and cosmetic needs related to her disease and its treatment. Reach to Recovery volunteers are breast cancer survivors who are carefully selected and trained by the American Cancer Society. They may visit a patient personally or by telephone at the discretion and convenience of the patient. Current information is provided to enable the patient, in consultation with her physician, to arrive at a treatment decision. The patient may request a Reach to Recovery visit at any point in her breast cancer experience. The volunteer will also supply a temporary breast form and information regarding a more permanent prosthesis and surgical reconstruction if desired.

THE WIG BANK

Patients often tell the volunteers that the diagnosis of cancer was overwhelming, but dealing with their hair loss was devastating!!

The Wig Bank volunteers try to help the patients through this difficult time by providing a complementary wig, turban, or other head covering. Patients are fitted with their wigs in a private, homey setting. They are encouraged to select a style and color close to their own in order to feel as "normal" as possible.

LOOK GOOD...FEEL BETTER

This program is a national service which teaches female cancer patients beauty techniques to enhance their appearance and self-image during chemotherapy and radiation treatments. The program is a joint effort of the Cosmetic, Toiletry and Fragrance Association, the National Cosmetology Association, and the American Cancer Society.

Each group session is led by trained beauty professionals and consists of up to 12 women. Through practical hands-on experience, women learn a 12-step makeup program. They are shown beauty tips about wigs, hats, turbans, and scarves. Each participant receives a complimentary box of make-up containing items used in the program.

This is an excellent opportunity for patients to interact with other women in treatment. Frequently, the new-found friendships continue long after the session ends!!

BREAST PROSTHESIS

Frequently, patients who have mastectomy will need to have either a temporary or permanent breast prosthesis. While the ACS encourages their patients to go through their insurance companies for breast prosthesis, the Information Center has established a program whereby uninsured breast cancer patients may be fitted with a complementary prosthesis and/or bra.

ROAD TO RECOVERY

This program of the American Cancer Society provides free transportation to and from physician offices, chemotherapy and radiation treatments. Patients are transported in American Cancer Society vans or in private automobiles by specially trained volunteers.

LENDING LIBRARY

Many educational books and videos are available for patients and their families. An assortment of light comedy videos help relieve pain and anxiety for patients during their recovery. Man has long declared laughter to be the best medicine. With an accurate understanding of the disease process and the available community resources, patients and families become more active participants in the diagnosis, treatment, and rehabilitation process. This enables them to cope more effectively with the stress associated with their disease.

This is the goal of the AMERICAN CANCER SOCIETY INFORMATION CENTER. (*See* Resources).

Chapter 28
PLASTIC SURGERY

After God created Adam, He looked around and said:
"I think we need a woman, to share his grassy bed."
So He took out one of Adam's ribs and in a thunderstorm
The rest is history, as we know He made the female form.

I guess we must consider Him the primal Plastic Surgeon.
Working with almost nothing, he created modern woman.
For many centuries doctors have repaired and changed our looks
They've written all about it and we have their ancient books.

And now we are indebted to these fine aesthetic draftsmen
They change or reconstruct the breast, they're anatomic craftsmen.
(But I must add whoever named 'em, was a little drastic,
They do a lot of surgery, but they never do use plastic.)

The primary focus on surgical treatment of breast disease is basically twofold. First and foremost is to eradicate the disease process as best possible with the least amount of physical deformity. When dealing with benign disease, there is usually a great deal of latitude in choosing a surgical procedure which will eliminate the disease because it is not so important to completely eradicate the process such as a benign lump (fibroadenoma or intraductal papilloma) or draining an abscess or aspirating a cyst. If the first procedure is not sufficient, a second may be needed, but there is no life-threatening problem involved. In general, the treatment of benign disease by the general surgeon is not very deforming, and the services of a trained plastic and reconstructive surgeon are not needed. The treatment of the breast for elective cosmetic procedures has come of age in the United States with the major procedures being augmentation mammoplasty (enlargement of the breast), reduction mammoplasty (reduction in size of the breast), and procedures which combine these two for the treatment of ptosis or sagging of the breasts which occurs as women get older, have weight gain or loss, and after pregnancy. Large painful breasts are often very distressful to young women, and may need reduction on a non-cosmetic and insurance-covered basis because of shoulder and back pain, and this requires a skillful plastic surgeon to evaluate and properly correct the situation. We will discuss each of these procedures as this chapter progresses.

But we must consider another and perhaps a more critical area of surgical approach to the breast, and that is in the treatment of cancer. It is important to emphasize that of primary importance is the completeness of the surgical eradication of the cancer. Although we have abbreviated the surgery in the past one hundred years from radical Halsted mastectomy to modified mastectomy to lumpectomy with axillary dissection (or with sentinel node biopsy) followed by radiation to the remaining breast, the procedure which is done must be complete enough to eradicate the tumor cells so as to give the greatest chance for cure. While cosmesis (getting a good cosmetic result) is of major importance, it must play a secondary role to the primary objective of eliminating the cancer. As has been described, we may sometimes have to do mastectomies because of the diffuse nature of the cancer or the large size of the tumor, and this leaves a woman with a major deformity in the chest which has grave emotional, psychological, cosmetic, social, and physical side effects. It is after these procedures that the plastic surgeon is called in to reconstruct the breast to the most cosmetically pleasing state possible. Women should understand that no surgeon will be able to give them back a completely normal appearing breast. The reconstructed breast will look different, feel different, and have surgical scars as a result of the procedure. But the overall result will be a tremendous improvement over the postmastectomy condition. Most women are able to wear bathing suits, normal dresses with adequate cleavage and balance to the other breast to enjoy a normal social life. The deformity of the breast when seen unclothed is a great improvement from the mastectomy condition, and a woman will usually be able to resume a normal sexual life after reconstruction. It is strongly recommended that all women with cancer have interaction with group therapy and appropriate counseling to help them through the transition, and after mastectomy and reconstruction, it must be emphasized that psychosocial support plays an important role. There are, of course, many women who don't opt for reconstruction and may accept their physical status very well. But later in this chapter we want to focus on those procedures which are now available for reconstructing the breast.

We will divide the chapter into two sections:

1. The treatment of benign disease such as mammary hypertrophy (enlarged breast), cosmetic augmentation and reduction mammoplasties, and ptosis procedures, and reconstruction after elective prophylactic mastectomies in very high-risk women (we'll talk more about the indications), and

2. The reconstruction of the breast after surgical removal of the breast for cancer.

The first part I will discuss, and the second, I will defer to the expertise of Plastic and Reconstructive Surgeon, Dr. Malcolm Paul.

Benign Disease

The most common procedure is the augmentation mammoplasty, usually done on an outpatient basis under general anesthesia. The procedure consists of placing a saline-filled sac behind the breast and under the pectoralis major muscle. Depending on your choice and the expertise of your surgeon, the incisions may be inframammary (under the breast), peri-areolar (around part of the areola) or axillary (in the axilla or armpit). The scar is usually very small but will depend to a large degree on your own scar formation. You will be given ample information prior to the surgery, and select an appropriate breast cup size after discussion with the surgeon. The major complications are bleeding, unequal size, change in position, and rarely skin loss or nipple and areolar loss or partial loss. It is a very common surgery, and complications should be fairly rare. Those that do occur are usually correctable with a second procedure with an excellent cosmetic result. A later complication is development of encapsulation around the implant secondary to the body's reaction to the "foreign material'. Some women have soft breasts after their augmentation while others develop very firm, uncomfortable scarring, and encapsulation around the "sac" which may require surgical intervention or even removal of the implants. After the surgery, you will probably have a drain in placed for a few days, and will be advised about minimal chest wall movement, and precautions about injuring the chest wall. There may also be some ecchymosis around the breast, and the incision which will resolve over several weeks. Your surgeon will give you instructions regarding breast massage, appropriate bras, and activities after the augmentation. Figure 52 shows the breast after the augmentation. Remember, the excellence of the surgery will be directly related to the expertise and training of your plastic surgeon. Many can do the procedure; not so many can do it well This procedure is usually considered purely cosmetic and will usually not be covered by your insurance.

NORMAL BREAST   AFTER IMPLANT

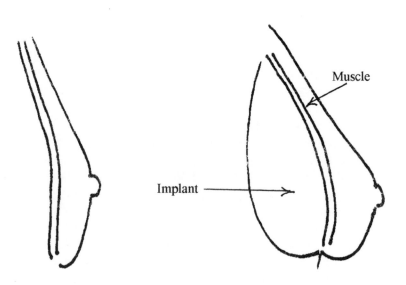

Figure 52. NORMAL BREAST AFTER IMPLANT.

Straightforward Reduction Mammoplasty is done on women with large painful breasts or with back pain or cosmetic deformity because of the large size. Depending on the situation, it may be covered by insurance.

Malignant Disease

When a radical procedure is done to eliminate a cancer, one of the primary concerns is minimizing the amount of physical distortion caused by the surgeon. The psychological effects of the cancer and the surgery will be addressed by the clinical psychologist, the surgeon, the primary physician, and the oncologists, but the Plastic Surgeon plays a key role is restoring a semblance of normalcy to the woman's life. Dr. Malcolm Paul has lectured and taught nationally and internationally. He has always been ready to get involved in this most delicate of situations when called upon by the surgeon or oncologist. His contribution is an excellent discourse on breast reconstruction after mastectomy.

Breast Reconstruction After Mastectomy

At the outset, let me say that breast reconstruction after mastectomy for cancer is fully covered by insurance. Over the past several years, there has been an increasing awareness of the various options available to women seeking breast reconstruction after cancer surgery. There also is an increasing acceptance of both the psychological and physical benefits that breast reconstruction provides, and younger and healthier patients with an excellent chance for a cure appear to be ideal candidates for reconstruction. Many women are candidates for less involved surgical therapies for breast cancer, which may include lumpectomy with sampling of axillary nodes followed by radiation therapy or even removing a quadrant or one-forth of the breast with associated lymph nodes. These patients often do not require reconstruction of the breast depending upon the size of the breast and what the opposite breast looks like. Some patients require insertion of a breast implant to fill out the area that was removed by a less aggressive type removal of breast tissue. Other patients may simply require the opposite breast to be adjusted in terms of volume to match the breast that has had only a section removed for cancer treatment.

It is the patient who requires a modified radical mastectomy that typically presents for breast reconstruction. A modified radical mastectomy is a procedure wherein the entire breast is removed including the nipple and areola and a sampling of axillary lymph nodes is performed. Many patients that have this procedure performed can be reconstructed at the time of the mastectomy in one of several ways. This is called Immediate Breast Reconstruction.

The options for immediate breast reconstruction include the insertion of a tissue expander. This involves placement of a breast implant, which is basically a silicone envelope, which is placed beneath the chest muscle in a deflated position. After the breast incision has healed, which is usually about 10 days to two weeks after surgery, the implant can be gradually inflated by inserting a needle beneath the skin and injecting sterile saltwater solution to gradually expand the implant. This has the effect of gradually increasing the size of the breasts to match the ideal size that the patient and the surgeon agree to. After a period of several weeks of expansion, the patient is ready for perhaps the most ideal autogenous reconstruction which is the use of the abdominal tissue for reconstruction. In this case, the skin and fatty tissue of the lower abdomen that would normally be discarded in a tummy tuck is left connected to the blood vessels and rotated underneath the skin of the chest and brought up to the mastectomy defect to reconstruct the breast as it was prior to the mastectomy. At the same time the abdominal skin is tightened as are the underlying muscles to create a flat tummy with a single transverse scar above the hairline and a scar around the umbilicus. This type of reconstruction is ideal when available since it allows a true Robin Hood principle. In this case, the abdomen that is rich in skin and fatty tissue in many women will give up its excess to provide it to the poor, which in this case is the breast that is deficient in skin and fatty tissue due to the mastectomy.

This is a win-win type of situation wherein the breast is reconstructed with one's own tissue, creating a soft, natural match to the opposite breast, and at the same time the abdomen becomes more youthful with a better contour and flattening due to the result of removing the excess skin and fatty tissues and tightening the muscle.

In some cases, the abdominal skin and fatty tissue can be completely removed from the abdominal wall, and the blood vessels that keep this tissue alive can be connected directly to blood vessels in the underarm area to nourish the tissues without having to pass the tissues from the abdomen to the chest through a tunnel. This is a highly specialized procedure that is the least commonly performed of the reconstructed procedures.

In summary, immediate breast reconstruction includes either the use of a tissue expander which is placed temporarily to be followed by removal of the filling valve thereby leaving the implant in place or replacing the implant with a permanent saltwater filled or gel filled implant. Other options, as mentioned above, include use of autogenous tissue such as skin and muscle from the back with an implant or the use of the abdominal wall tissues to reconstruct the breasts. Typically, about three months after the reconstruction is completed, the nipple areola complex is reconstructed. This involves utilizing local segments of skin and fatty tissue on the reconstructed breasts that are raised as small flaps to assimilate the appearance of the opposite nipple. A skin graft taken from the lower abdomen or inner thigh is used in a doughnut fashion around the nipple flaps for reconstructing the areola to match the opposite side. Typically, tattooing of the reconstructed nipple areola complex is required for color match and this can be done as an office or outpatient procedure.

This second major type of breast reconstruction is termed Delayed Reconstruction. This means that the reconstruction is not performed at the time of the mastectomy but rather performed at some time subsequent to this. One might ask, "Why would not all of the reconstructions be done at the time of the mastectomy?" In some cases, the tissues at the time are not amenable to reconstruction due to such factors as excessive weight of the patient, smoking history, etc. In this case, it may be more prudent to allow the tissues to heal and then develop a pocket for the breast implant or reconstruct the breast with the options mentioned above at a later date. Many women chose to have the reconstruction done at the time of the mastectomy as it avoids a second operating room session with the requirements of a second anesthesia session as well. The same procedures mentioned above can be utilized. There are patients, however, who undergo delayed reconstruction and merely require the insertion of a permanent implant rather than requiring a tissue expander since the tissues have already healed, and there is a very low risk of any problem with the wound healing if a permanent implant is inserted rather than going through the stage of tissue expansion. Tissue expansion is required when the mastectomy and reconstruction are performed at the same time since the tissues tend to be tight and will not heal well if a permanent implant were inserted behind this fresh tissue at the same time.

Although there have been many reports of excellent to good cosmetic results after conservative procedures such as lumpectomy or quadrantectomy and radiation therapy without reconstruction, there are a number of problems with reconstructing a breast after these procedures when it is required. These tissues typically that have been radiated do show postoperative radiation fibrosis which makes reconstruction difficult and also reconstruction must be performed carefully so as not to interfere with clinical or radiographic detection of locally recurrent disease in these patients that have an almost 10% risk of recurrent disease. Many of these patients may eventually undergo a total mastectomy either because the local disease could not be controlled or there is a significant deformity from the conservative treatment or because it was difficult to follow the breast over a long period of time for local recurrence. In these cases, it is more difficult to reconstruct the breast because of prior radiation changes as mentioned above, and typically these patients do best with use of autologous tissue such as using their abdominal wall tissue for reconstruction or utilizing the tissue from the back with placement of an implant as well.

Obviously, each case must be managed individually based upon the clinical findings and the close working relationship between the general surgeon and reconstructive plastic surgeon. It is important to mention that breast reconstruction at the time of mastectomy or in the delayed mode in no way interferes with the future detection of recurrent breast cancer, nor does the reconstruction in any way increase the chance of recurrent breast cancer.

Refinements in the techniques of breast reconstruction at the time of or subsequent to mastectomy have continued to evolve over the past 20 years. This evolution has produced wonderfully satisfying results for patient and physician alike. Women can be made whole again and be made to feel feminine both in and out of their clothing. There is enormous psychological benefit to feeling normal and being able to look in a mirror and feel good about one's self is essential for a sense of well being.

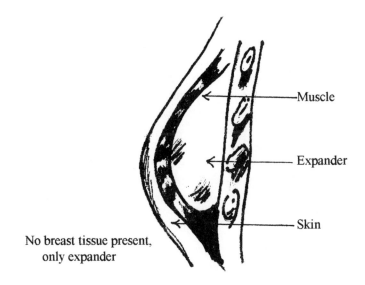

No breast tissue present, only expander

Muscle

Expander

Skin

Figure 53. FIRST STAGE OF RECONSTRUCTIVE SURGERY.

Chapter 29
VIEWS
FROM A MAMMOGRAPHY TECHNOLOGIST

I'm getting my mammogram today
I couldn't be much droller.
It seems like someone wants to play
As if they're a small steam roller.

I have no doubt it was a man
Who devised this medieval torture.
A woman would never, ever plan
A test that would so contort her.

I hope some day they need a test
For men, (and you know where)
I'll be the one, as you have guessed,
To design it fair and square!

T he primary reason I'm not writing this chapter is because I'm not a woman and haven't undergone the indelicacy of having my breasts squashed between two metal plates during a mammographic examination. The second reason I'm not writing the chapter is because I have at hand the expertise of a mammography technologist, Lynn McBride, with many years of experience, a warm and charming personality, and an ability to relate well to women patients to set them at ease while undergoing this exam. Her chapter on mammography is comprehensive, and a pleasant read, to boot.

There's a lot of mystery surrounding mammography, and most women never ask and never have all their questions answered. I have attempted here to answer what you'd like to know to make the best of your mammogram exam, as seen through the eyes of one of our finest technologists.

Where To Go For A Mammogram?

Go to an FDA (Federal Drug Administration) accredited facility. (The certificate should be posted in the waiting room--if not, ask for it.)

What Do I Need To Know When Scheduling My Mammogram Appointment?

Schedule between 1-2 weeks after your period when your breasts are less tender or when you know your breasts are less tender. Tell the scheduler if you've had implants Exams with implants take a special method and need extra time to do.

Anytime you go to a new facility, whether for routine mammogram (or ultrasound), or for further workup, bring your films from the previous facility. Without your previous films, it's kind of like building a house without a foundation. You will less likely have additional films taken (and the technologist can anticipate technical adjustments if she can see your previous films before x-raying your breasts). There is also less chance for you to be called back for additional films.

Comparing previous mammograms, besides being required as part of a facility's accreditation, is one of the best tools we have to make sure your breasts are healthy. Keep track of your mammogram films Facilities are required to keep them for seven years (and this is a federal law so even out-of-state facilities come under this ruling). Usually, all it takes to request your films is a written note with your name and birth date, and the address to where you want them sent. Give facilities enough time to mail them to your new facility (most places send these films by mule train--or so it seems). Some places do charge for this service, while most don't. It's still worth the money because if we can't get your previous mammogram, the radiologist may ask for additional views, which you'll pay for both financially and physically (ouch!); so the effort to retrieve your previous films seems a lot easier than a more extensive exam. Of course, if you always go to he same facility, you won't have to mess around with this issue, but then, insurance change, you move, or maybe you don't like the facility; for whatever reason, you may not get to come back. Be sure in writing for previous films or just filling out your patient information sheets to print clearly and make sure you keep your address and phone number current. This is very important (You'd think with the technologist being able to read a doctor's handwriting they could read all sorts of writing--well, yes they're pretty good, but it's important to be able to get a hold of you for additional views).

In Preparation For The Appointment

Bring something to read, needlework, a crossword puzzle, homework, darn your husband's socks, whatever You may not have a long wait but this can reduce anxiety. Though everyone is different, some people (we do have males on rare occasions) have no problem with the mammogram appointment, but it does seem to be the most anxiety-inducing exam we go through. If you have concerns, let the technologist know. She can help. The technologists are trained to help patients with the stress of the exam but she does have limita-tions. Sometimes personalities don't mesh well, and you can ask for another technologist. Fortunately, this doesn't happen often. Some technologists talk to their patients during the exam, but sometimes a woman doesn't want to talk, and we also have technologists who work without talking. It may be a better match. Bring a sweater. Waiting in those mammogram gowns and being nervous can really cause chills, and summertime does help—but the air conditioning is on!

Do not wear lotion, oil, powder or deodorant under your arms or on your breasts. Powder and deodorant can imitate microcalcifications which can cause unnecessary film repeats or additional film workup. As far as lotion or oil is concerned, the technician can't get on film what she can't grasp, and she may miss some breast tissue if she can't get an adequate hold of the tissue.

During Your Appointment

It seems impossible to ask that you relax during the exam, but you'll be able to follow the technician's instructions better. A tense patient has tense chest muscles that can hold back the breast tissue from being examined. If the technician starts taking additional films, know that most of the time these films show there is nothing to be worried about. Some cases are easier than others so don't try to rush the doctor into a reading. And don't try to search the technologist's face or try to trick her into revealing what you think she knows, and is secretly holding back from telling you. Don't get angry with her. Don't tell her you don't think her facility is doing a good job or any other "traps" to find an answer. Let her concentrate on doing a good job, and then at the end of the examination see if you can get results from the radiologist. A facility doing a good job may not be able to give an instant answer.

Same if you are called back for additional views or for an ultrasound. Most of the time, these additional views will show there is nothing to worry about, but they are very important to do. The exam is not complete until the recommended extra views have been read. In many facilities, the radiologist will give you the results at the end of the procedure. If you have questions--ask!

There is an early followup mammogram method used if there is no previous mammogram available (remember the importance of keeping track of your mammograms) or if the exam was your first-time mammogram (baseline mammogram). Looking for changes is one of the ways the radiologist uses to look for any problems (these can be very subtle), and having previous films allows him to do this.

Do not read periodical articles on mammography and breast health and accept them as gospel. There are many fine articles but there are also many misleading ones. The library, the American Cancer Society, and other sources listed in the reference section of this book have many good articles to read on breast health. And please ask your technician any questions about mammography matters. There are many good community lectures conducted by physicians and other health care professionals from the larger hospitals in your area, and most of these are free (that wonderful word!).

Remember that we want to find any abnormality at an early stage. You have read many times (even in this book) about the three things to do to increase your chance of finding a very early stage breast cancer:

- Clinical Exam by a Doctor
  Age 20-39: Every 3 years; 40 years and up: Every year
- Mammography

35-40 years: Baseline exam (there are differing opinions about this)
40 years and up: Every year
- Breast Self Exam
Age: Every month starting at age 20

There's always something in the news about a better machine for mammography. Unfortunately the old "squishmaster" has yet to be replaced by anything as effective.

Regarding the concerns about the radiation received from a mammogram--it's very low dose, and there is no data to support any harmful effects (of course, care should be taken if you are pregnant).

Chapter 30
ANESTHESIA

Be sure before you operate that I am sleeping soundly,
I'm really very frightened and I mean this quite profoundly.
If I wake up and you're not done, I don't know what I'd do,
But if it happens be assured I'll do the same to you.

I think I'm getting sleepy now, my head is turning fuzzy
My eyes are getting blurry and my ears are kind of buzzy.
You say you never ever fail to get some one asleep,
But I'm the exception to the rule, I'll never......

Anesthesia is a frightening word, but the people who do this work are anything but frightening. In general, these physicians are usually the most relaxed, tranquil, reassuring physicians you will ever meet. And although they give medications and gases to make you fall asleep, it is probably not appropriate to say that they are physicians who spend their working day passing gas.

As a surgeon, I am constantly relying on their expertise in the management of my patients, and although the anesthesia for breast surgery may not be as complex as in other procedures, to the patient, it's a major thing to be put to sleep for any reason. Anesthesiologist, Dr. Sara Myla, is trained as a general and cardiac (open heart procedures) anesthesiologist, and is well aware of the various risks and anxieties which her patients undergo. As with all good anesthesiologists, she reviews the patient's records, examines them, and discusses the type of anesthetic she will be administering. She is a compassionate, caring, and skilled physician, and she had written an insightful chapter on Anesthesia and Breast Surgery.

ANESTHESIA AND BREAST SURGERY

Most of you are getting over the initial shock of the diagnosis, fear of unknown and worry. As anesthesiologists, we do understand the difficult time that you are going through, and try our level best to make your anesthetic experience as pleasant as possible.

What does your anesthesiologist do while you are under his or her care? It starts with pre-op evaluation and treatment, consultation with the surgical team, intra-op pain control, monitoring and medical management, post-anesthetic evaluation and treatment and finally, discharge from the post-anesthesia recovery unit.

Depending on the extent of surgery the decision will be made to do it as an outpatient (same day) procedure or as an inpatient procedure. Except for a radical procedure most of the surgical procedures on the breast are done on an outpatient basis.

MOST FREQUENTLY ASKED QUESTIONS

1. What is same day surgery?

Same day surgical procedure is one where the patient can come to the hospital, have surgery and go home all on the same day. New, safe, short-acting anesthetic medications and sophisticated monitoring devices enable us to allow you to go home and recuperate in the comfort of your own home, and often avoid costs which insurance companies might not cover.

2. Can I choose my anesthesiologist?

Yes You can choose your anesthesiologist based on personal recommendation from a friend or based on your personal experience. However, you need to make that choice known to the surgeon earlier on so that arrangements can be made to honor your request. Usually your surgeon may refer you to a particular anesthesiologist and if for any reason you are not comfortable with the choice you may request a different anesthesiologist.

3. What is pre-admission testing?

During pre-admission testing, blood tests, ECG, and x-rays will be obtained. This testing enables us to do necessary further work-up and consultation if an abnormality is detected so that we do not have to delay your surgery.

4. What is the purpose of the pre-operative interview?

Pre-operative evaluation gives you an opportunity to discuss your medical history, various anesthetic options and their risks, and pertinent questions of concern with your anesthesiologist. In some instances, this interview can be done over the phone the night before surgery. You should bring a list of all medications that you take on a regular basis or have taken recently with you to the pre-op interview or testing area. Some of these medications can alter the response of patients to anesthetics; some may even cause adverse drug reactions. You may be advised to discontinue taking certain medications since they can cause life-threatening problems under anesthesia. This information combined with laboratory data from your tests is the basis upon which many anesthetic decisions are made. During this interview, do not forget to notify your anesthesiologist of any allergies that you may have (medications and latex). If you have not met your anesthesiologist during your pre-operative interview, you will meet him or her immediately before your surgery at which time a limited physical exam will be performed to evaluate the status of the heart, lungs and airway.

5. Why do I have to discontinue herbal medications?

Most patients believe that herbal medications are natural and safe and continue to take them through the surgery. Just because a medicine is called natural or herbal, does not mean that it is completely safe. Most of these products are very potent with serious adverse effects on the heart and the circulation. Following are a few commonly used herbal products and their effects:

St. John's Wort: This medication is used to treat anxiety, depression, and sleep disorders. It is reported to prolong and intensity the effects of narcotics and anesthetic agents.

Gingko Biloba: It is used to improve their memory and blood circulation. It is known to reduce platelets, which are necessary for blood to clot formation and prevent bleeding.

Gin Seng: Most popular herbal product, believed to boost vitality and energy. It is associated with episodes of high blood pressure and rapid heart rate.

The American Society of Anesthesiologists advises patients to stop taking these herbal medications up to two to three weeks prior to surgery. If there is not enough time to stop, bring the product in its original container and show it to the physicians involved in your care, especially the anesthesiologist who has the critical responsibility for your welfare when you are under anesthesia.

6. Why can't I eat or drink before my anesthesia?

As a general rule, you should refrain from eating or drinking after midnight or eight hours prior to surgery to allow your stomach to be empty. Most anesthetics suspend your normal reflexes so that your body's automatic defenses may not be working. For example, your lungs are normally protected from objects such as undigested food from entering them. This natural protection does not occur while you are anesthetized. For your safety, you may be advised to fast before surgery. You may be told to take some of your medications with a sip of water. It is very important to follow these instructions for your safety, failing which, it may be necessary to postpone your surgery.

7. Why are so many questions asked about my past and present medical conditions?

Anesthesia affects your entire body so it is important for anesthesiologists to know as much information about you as possible. Remember that your anesthesiologist is responsible for your medical care during the entire course of the surgery; therefore, it is important to know exactly what medical problems you have and what medications that you have taken recently since they may effect your response to anesthesia. You also need to inform your anesthesiologist about any hard drug or alcohol usage and past anesthetic experiences.

8. Why do I need to talk about my personal habits such as drinking and smoking?

Cigarettes and alcohol can affect your body just as strongly as any other medically prescribed drugs that you may be taking. Because of their various effects on your lungs, heart, liver and blood, to name a few, cigarette and alcohol consumption can change the way an anesthetic drug will work during surgery, so it is very crucial to let your anesthesiologist know about your consumption of the above.

Cigarette smoking causes constant irritation of breathing tubes (bronchi) and air sacs (alveoli) in the lungs. Oxygen goes out of little sacs and into the blood, while carbon dioxide flows into them to be breathed out through bronchial tubes. Smoking causes narrowing of these tubes and buildup of mucus which works like a road block in the smaller bronchi and oxygen cannot reach air sacs, so blood passing through these blocked air sacs will not pickup oxygen, so not as much oxygen will reach tissues as it should. In addition to the above, Carbon Monoxide in the cigarette smoke binds to the hemoglobin in the blood, which carries oxygen throughout your body. Since carbon monoxide binds to hemoglobin 200 times stronger than oxygen, oxygen availability to the tissues is compromised because of inability of oxygen to be released freely to the tissues.

Quit smoking cigarettes, as far in advance as possible. If you are unable to do so, at least decrease the number of cigarettes you smoke each day. Try not to smoke on the night before surgery. All of these measures will decrease the irritation to the air passages. For those that suffer from nicotine withdrawal, your anesthesiologist may be able to give you a mild sedative in order to help.

The same applies to the so-called "street drugs"--marijuana, cocaine, amphetamine, etc. Though you may be reluctant to discuss such issues, it is worth remembering that such discussions are entirely confidential between you and your physician. Your anesthesiologists' only interest in these subjects is to provide you with the safest anesthesia possible so in this case, honesty is definitely the best policy, and the safest one.

9. What is the purpose of pre-operative medication?
Pre-operative medication provides:
- Anxiety relief
- Sedation
- Pain Relief
- Dryness of airway
- Smooth induction of anesthesia

- Reduction of stomach secretions
- Decreases post-operative vomiting

10. How do anesthesiologist determines the Dosage of medications?
- Patient's age and weight
- ASA physical status
- Level of anxiety
- Tolerance to depressant drugs
- Previous adverse experience with pre-medications
- Inpatient vs. outpatient
- Emergency vs. elective surgery

11. What are the commonly used pre-operative medications?
- Anti-Anxiety medications
  - Midazolam
  - Diazepam
  - Lorazepam
- Analgesics
  - Morphine
  - Demerol
  - Fentanyl
- Gastrokinetic
  - Metoclopramide
- Anti-emetic
  - Droperidol
  - Metoclopramide
- Anti-Sialogogue (mouth-drying agents)
  - Atropine
  - Scopolamine
  - Glycopyrrolate

12. What are the types of anesthesia?
General anesthesia
During general anesthesia, you are unconscious, not aware of any stimuli. Usually anesthetic gases along with oxygen are inhaled through a breathing mask or tube and other medications are given to the patient through the intravenous catheter which is already in place.

You are carefully monitored and the length and level of anesthesia is calculated and constantly adjusted with great precision. At the end, your anesthesiologist reverses the process causing you will regain awareness.

Conscious Sedation

During conscious sedation, you are given medications through the IV line which make you drowsy as well as relieve your pain. The surgeon also injects a local anesthetic to make the area of incision numb. Under conscious sedation you will respond appropriately to commands and maintain an unassisted and patent airway.

Local Anesthesia

During local anesthesia, you remain awake while your surgeon injects medication at the site of incision and numbs the area.

13. Can I request the type of anesthesia?

Yes After reviewing the extent of surgery, prior medical history, etc., your Anesthesiologist discusses your anesthetic options with you and you may choose one over the other if you wish.

14. During surgery what does my anesthesiologist do?

In the OR, your anesthesiologist will monitor your critical life functions such as breathing, heart rate, rhythm, blood pressure, body temperature and body fluid balance as they are affected by the surgery being performed. He assesses your medical condition continuously, controls pain and your level of consciousness to make conditions ideal for a safe and successful surgery. The anesthetic needs of each patient are different. Your anesthesiologist takes you and your medical condition into consideration, and tailors the anesthetics especially for you.

15. What can I expect after the operation and before I go home?

You will be taken to the post-anesthesia care unit, commonly known as the recovery room. Your heart rhythm, blood pressure, breathing rate and pattern and other vital functions are monitored very closely by specially trained nurses. It is possible that you will experience pain, nausea, vomiting, high or low blood pressure, cardiac rhythmic irregularities, inadequate oxygenation and inadequate ventilation. You will be appropriately treated and managed under the guidance of anesthesiologists.

Depending on your prior medical condition, several situations can arise. For example, if you have a prior history of hypertension poorly controlled by medications or you are non-compliant with medications, you may experience fluctuations in blood pressure, high as well as low. You may also experience heart rate and rhythm abnormalities. But no matter the situation, your anesthesiologist should be able to appropriately treat the situation. This is the reason why it is very important to let your anesthesiologist know about your prior medical as well as medication history.

16. Will I have any side effects?

Your anesthesiologist administers some medication towards the avoidance of nausea and pain in the post-operative period. Your discomfort should be tolerable but do not expect to be totally pain-free. In case you experience pain in the post-anesthesia recovery unit, you will receive appropriate pain medications.

17. When will I be able to go home?

Based on the extent of surgery, your ability to recover from anesthesia and your hospital policy, you should be able to go home anywhere from one to four hours after surgery. In some cases, it may be necessary to stay overnight.

It is important to pre-arrange your ride home after surgery since your coordination and various reflexes may be impaired for at least 24 hours or more, making normal activities, let alone driving, very difficult.

18. What can I expect after going home?

You will tend to experience drowsiness. On the other hand, some patients experience muscle aches, sore throats, dizziness and headaches. Nausea can also be expected while vomiting is less common. These effects will go down rapidly at times hours following surgery but can also take several days before they completely disappear.

For 24 hours after your anesthesia:
- Refrain from consuming alcohol and non-prescription medications
- Try not to drive or operate dangerous machinery
- Try not to make important decisions

Follow the instructions given by the surgical facility. If you have any questions, feel free to contact your anesthesiologist.

In the days following surgery, you might get a telephone call or questionnaire to mail back inquiring about your surgical and anesthetic experience. Please voice your opinions. This enables us to provide the best care possible to our patients.

19. Where can I get access to more information?
American Society of Anesthesiologists is a great organization to get further information. Thanks for their continuing efforts to educate the public regarding "Person behind the mask" (Anesthesiologist) and what they do. Incidentally some of the information in this chapter is obtained from them.
- Directories/References on the Internet
- *www.achoo.com* Internet health care directory
- *www.nlm.nih.com* National Library of Medicine/Medline Search
- General Links on the Internet
- *www.ama-assn.org* American Medical Association
- *www.medicalert.org* Medic Alert
- Publications
- New England Journal of Medicine

Chapter 31
OPERATING ROOM NURSE

You say your surgeon's charming, a gentleman and more,
But something seems to happen when he clears the OR door.
You say that he's an angel, but to us he's fallen down,
To you he very serious, to us a raving clown.

He treats you like a gentle soul, he treats us like soul food,
You say he's always kind and sweet, to us he's always rude.
I sometimes think the air in here must have a strange pollutant
It changes your dear surgeon into some demented mutant.

But we're well trained and tolerant and do just what he pleases,
Because we know he saves lives and will stamp out all diseases.
And if you really think that's true, I really want to weep.
Why do you think the surgeons insist we put you all to sleep?

If any patient saw her professed "god" in cap and gown,
Yelling, throwing instruments, and working with a frown,
She'd never let him operate, much less do an exam
She'd realize her surgeon is a transcendental sham.

Surgeons are just frustrated that they can't be private plumbers,
Who get paid well and drive around in manly cars like Hummers.
Instead the surgeon vents his ire (and certainly not his purse)
On the next available whipping girl, the operating room nurse.

Okay I've been a little cruel, they're not as bad as that
Sometimes they buy us pizzas or will liposuck our fat.
I even know a certain doc who'd take out my gallbladder
(And when I told him it was out, he said it didn't matter.)

But there are a few kind souls who walk unblemished
through our door.
They're usually young and haven't learned why real lions roar.
And hopefully we'll find that in this new fresh generation,
The surgeons will behave and give the nurse due veneration.

I f you want to find out who's a good surgeon--ask the operating room nurse. Unfortunately, they're usually too polite to let you know, but they're the ones who watch the day in and day out functioning of the OR and know what's what. As surgeons, we usually just walk in and expect everything to be taken care of from the patients to the instruments. For this reason, I felt it would be a good idea to have one of our best surgical nurses give her own perspective of what goes on behind the operating room doors. I have worked with nurse, Carole Metcalf, for several years and have watched her work up to becoming supervisor as well as an excellent nurse first assistant on any and all of my surgeries. I think you will enjoy her discussion of The Masked Strangers.

THE MASKED STRANGERS

As a breast cancer patient, you will probably need surgery sometime in the course of your treatment. Facing the "masked strangers" behind the double doors of the operating room can be a frightening and overwhelming experience. Being informed and involved in all aspects of your care promotes trust, and provides the opportunity to participate in decisions regarding your care with confidence and realistic expectations. In this chapter, I would like to take the opportunity to describe what experiences you will encounter on your day of surgery.

INTRODUCTION OF THE MASKED STRANGERS
It may seem you are you are encountering an overwhelming number of "masked strangers" as you enter the surgical suite. By learning who they are and what they do, you will have a better understanding of the role they will play in your care. I would like to "introduce" you to some of the operating room staff that will

probably participate in your procedure and briefly describe their functions.

• TRANSPORTATION ASSISTANT

The first person you may encounter in the lovely scrub outfit will probably be the attendant that will transport you to the surgical department. Usually identified by the slightly dated, but still functional, term of orderly, he will greet you, confirm your name, matches your chart and name band, and provide you a private vehicle (usually a gurney, but perhaps a wheelchair) for your ride to the department.

• HOLDING AREA NURSE

No, this is not a nurse that will physically hold you, but rather the RN that will be in charge of your care in the minutes immediately prior to your procedure. The "holding area" serves the purpose of having the patients in the immediate vicinity prior to the actual start time of the procedure, where many last minute preparations are performed, and is an excellent place to have many important questions answered. If your procedure is done as an outpatient or in a same day surgery center, your admitting area may serve as your holding area and your discharge area as well.

• ANESTHESIOLOGIST

Fondly known to the OR team as the "gas passer", your anesthesiologist is a specialty trained physician whose participation in your procedure is of great importance. He will meet with you before your procedure (probably in the holding area) and discuss with you the many choices of anesthesia for your procedure. He will collaborate with your surgeon to provide the best combination of agents for the type of surgery you will be having and answer your questions regarding these choices. At this time, the anesthesiologist will want to discuss previous surgical procedures you have had, as well as the types of anesthesia and reactions you may have had during those procedures.

• OPERATING ROOM NURSES

Your procedure will require a minimum of two nurses. Your circulating nurse will greet you in the holding area, verify your identity and procedure, review your chart and accompany you through the entire procedure and into the recovery room. Your scrub nurse will be waiting for you the operating room and will work closely with your surgeon during the procedure providing the necessary supplies and equipment. Often seen in television and movie productions as the surgeon's "straight man" or vocal accompanist, the scrub nurse actually provides a much more somber role in real life, but be assured that it will be the duty of both nurses to provide hearty laughter for any jokes the surgeon may feel compelled to share with the staff during your surgery.

• YOUR SURGEON

While this may be the only member of the surgical team that you have a chance of recognizing on the day of your surgery, don't be surprised if, in fact, you do not recognize him until he speaks to you. The surgical garb can be very disguising, but a word of caution--if you find you had a hard time identifying your surgeon without his lab coat on, resist the urge to say, "Oh doctor, I didn't recognize you without your clothes!" or he may be tempted to say the same to you in return Depending upon the extent of your procedure, your surgeon may have one more assistant. The assistant may be a physician you already know, a physician your surgeon has chosen that you have not yet met, or a non-physician assistant such as an RNFA (Registered Nurse First Assistant). Your surgeon's assistant has been carefully selected and will be an important participant in your procedure.

• ADDITIONAL MASKED STRANGERS

The professionals listed above may be just a few of the many health care providers you are likely to encounter on a trip to the OR. Assistants, technicians, and support staff from other departments collaborate to provide care in a variety of ways for a variety of procedures. Be assured that all are working together to ensure your procedure goes as smoothly and comfortably as possible. If you are unsure of a person's identity or role, ask for clarification. It is your right to know who is providing your care.

THE SURGICAL EXPERIENCE:
WHAT TO EXPECT FROM START TO FINISH

You may think surgery would seem routine to the doctors and nurses who participate in operations on a daily basis, but be assured that they know it is far from routine to their patients. Every effort will be made to explain procedures and reassure you during your surgery, eliminating surprises and reducing anxiety wherever possible. I would like to describe to you in some detail exactly what would happen to you on the day of your surgery. Each operating room and each surgical team may have minor difference, but overall, patient's experiences are very similar.   In the holding area, attention is paid to assuring that everything is in order for your procedure. Your paper work will be inspected for completeness and you will be asked to verify your name, procedure, physician and allergies. The nurses will make sure you are properly dressed for your procedure, and unfortunately, that usually means you will be wearing only the very lovely patient gown. You will probably be given a paper cap to cover your hair, and will be asked to remove jewelry, prosthesis, denture, hair clips, and basically everything that can come off or out. Be sure to tell your nurse if you are feeling too cool, as the temperatures in the operating suite are usually more comfortable to the workers than to the scantily clad patients. She probably has a supply of warm blankets she will be happy to share with you. At this time, it is likely that you will be able to have a family member with you, which makes the waiting easier. It is during this time that the anesthesiologist will visit and assess your anesthesia needs. He will review your chart, ask questions regarding your general health, and may do a small physical exam. The anesthesiologist or the nurse will start an IV while you are in holding area. The IV will be your "pipeline", so to speak, for your anesthetic agents and is a very important part of your surgery. This is how you will receive many of your anesthetic agents as well as how you will receive fluid replacement. After your surgery, you will be able to receive pain medication via your IV eliminating painful injections. Usually the starting of the IV is relatively painless. Often a small amount of local anesthetic (numbing medication) is used and the introduction of the IV catheter can be barely felt. The catheter will be introduced into your vein and each patient has uniqueness in vein availability. I have often asked patients if they left their veins at home. Ideally, once the rubber tourniquet is placed around your arm, a perfect vein pops up, but this is sometimes not the case. Please be patient with the doctor or nurse that is trying to access your vein. It is not always easy to do, and they will want to be sure the IV is suitable for the administration of all your medications. Occasionally more than one attempt is necessary. If you have had venous puncture before and know exactly which of your veins is the perfect choice, feel free to let the nurse or doctor know. They are always hopeful to "get it on the first try" A special note here, though--your surgeon may prefer to have your IV on the opposite side of your surgical site, thus limiting the options. Once the IV is started and while you are still in the holding area, your anesthesiologist or the nurse may administer some "pre-op" medication which will provide a relaxing effect. This also may provide an amnesic effect, which means you may not actually remember anything beyond that point. The effect of the pre-op medication varies greatly from patient to patient. If you are feeling extremely nervous and apprehensive, discuss these feelings with your anesthesiologist at this time.

The circulating nurse from the OR will also meet you in the holding area and review your chart in much the same manner as those before you, repeating questions and in general making sure "all systems are go". Your family and friends will be shown where to wait, and as you are transported to the Operating Room you will still be awake, although you may not remember the transition at all. I have had many patients actually become very fearful at this point because they expected to be "out", and I reassure them that this is normal. Upon entry to the Operating Room, the staff will assist you in transferring to the surgical table and will attach monitors that will track your heartbeat, blood pressure and oxygen content. It is here and in the presence of the anesthesiologist that it is safest for you to actually be given anesthesia. Depending on your procedure, the decisions of your doctors, and your own choices, the type of anesthesia that is right for you will be administered at s time. The choice may have been local anesthesia, during which you will be awake or drowsy, or you may receive general and will become completely unconscious. If general is the choice, be aware that you may receive some oxygen first and feel one or more blood pressures being taken before you fall completely asleep. During this time, you may be having conversations with the staff and physicians around you, and feel free to continue to have any questions answered. We will all want you to feel as relaxed and comfortable as possible. More blankets are available at this time and you may be attached to additional equipment depending upon your procedure. You may also be aware of a "seat belt" being placed across your lap, as we enforce the seat belt law for this ride. As you feel yourself drifting off to sleep, think positive and happy thoughts. Your team surrounds you to take excellent care of you.

No matter how long your procedure takes, it will seem like no time at all to you, due to the anesthesia (that is if your choice was general anesthesia). You will actually begin your waking up process right in the operating room and will most likely be able to open your eyes and answer questions before you are taken to the recovery room, although it is usual to not remember at this stage. Your anesthesiologist and circulating nurse will transport you to the recovery room, and your surgeon will be there too. Your care will be transferred to the recovery room staff, which consists of registered nurses and their assistants who are expertly trained to deal with the post anesthesia patient. As you wake up, you will have oxygen delivered, probably by mask, and as you further awaken your need for that will diminish. You may feel cool and achy, and a variety of devices are available to warm you up--yours for the asking. I think that one of the most important things I can say to you for this stage of your procedure is to do the asking. Assessing the needs of the very drowsy patient can be difficult, so if at this time you are feeling discomfort of any kind, please ask for relief. The nurses will want to do all they can to provide you comfort. Sometime in the recovery room you may start to feel discomfort or pain from the procedure. Medication is available and will be administered through the IV, so please ask for it. This is a time of balance. Anesthetic agents are wearing off and the need for pain medication is beginning. Your description to the nurse of what you are feeling will help you receive the medication that is most safe and effective.

Your stay in the post anesthesia care unit (recovery room is a dated term now) will be tailored to your needs. From there you will be transported back to your room or the admission area you were in prior to your surgery. The nurses and staff will help you in your transfer and any information you need to take home with you will be provided in writing, and you will be given phone numbers to call if you have questions. Don't worry if you still feel a little groggy and feel you won't be able to remember all the important details. This is normal and there will be plenty of opportunity to review everything before you go home. Your surgeon will send home instructions specific to your procedure, and if your hospital stay continues your nurses have specific postoperative orders from your doctor to meet your needs.

ALL DRESSED UP

When your surgery is over, you will be "all dressed up". Well, at least you probably will have some sort of surgical dressing--anything from a Band-Aid to a full chest wrap. Instructions regarding the care of your dressing and when you should see your physician will be given to you. Prescriptions for medications and directions for their use will be given, as well as follow up numbers for any questions or concerns. I hope that by learning what lies ahead for your surgical experience, your entire visit to the operating room will be easier and more relaxing for you. We are not really strangers behind the surgical mask, but a team that wants to be known by you as caring participants in your road to recovery. Good luck to all of you.

Chapter 32
BREAST CANCER
PREVENTION

An ounce of prevention is definitely not worth the proverbial
pound of cure.
Whoever said that silly quote was obtuse and demure.
It's a far, far better thing you do, than you've ever done before,
Don't count your chickens before they hatch, they're worth
a whole lot more!

To be or not to be, and please look before you leap,
The cure is quite expensive, but prevention ain't so cheap.
He who laughs last, laughs best, 'tis true, but I'd rather laugh
first and last,
In order to find a prevention for cancer, I'll gladly run nude
in the grass.

But let bygones be bygones, for the best and worst of times,
They're working much harder on cancer, than I am on these
silly rhymes.
Suffice it to say that every day, there's always a new convention,
Where scientists meet, with hopes and ideas to find
a cancer prevention.

'Twas brillig and the slithy toves, Merry Christmas one and all;
When are they going to come up with the magic, so we won't have
cancer at all?
The writing's on the wall, they say, when will it go in a book?
If research's the answer, I'll give it a dollar, you betcha
by hook or by crook.

Now you'll hear all about some clinical trials (Tippecanoe

and Tyler too)
And if you pay attention you won't lose your head like
the wandering Nanki-Poo.
But pay close attention, Pay Peter, not Paul, and don't bring
your coals to Newcastle
And you will find pounds of prevention to get without
a significant hassle.

In conclusion I think that research in the pink will find
all the answers for cancer
In the meantime it's true that my message to you is only
a reader enhancer.
And if you have read this incredible nonsense, it should have been
time better spent
On doing some work in researching of cancer, at least that
would help pay the rent.

We have discussed different aspects of breast cancer prevention in several of the chapters, and I want to briefly collate all the information again for you under one heading. Some of you may ask whether there really are controllable factors influencing whether or not you will develop breast cancer. Let us look at the simple example of women living in Asian countries. The incidence of breast cancer among women is relatively low among Japanese women living in Japan. When they move to the United States, the incidence slowly rises until after several years their incidence equals that of the American born woman. Is it diet, work site, general carcinogens in the air, change in stress? Probably all of the above but we will try to make some sense of all the possible factors. Perhaps the greatest factors are the uncontrollable ones, the ones you carry, your genes, and as time goes by, more and more will be revealed to let us understand about how our internal body mechanisms cope with all the external factors, and perhaps some day we may even be able to manipulate genes so well that we can prevent cancer or significantly impact our chances of ever getting cancer. But let us now review those factors which we know about in the prevention of cancer.

First, we must review the information on nutrition and diet. Remember that, as with smoking, the deleterious effects of diet are apparently cumulative over many years. When you have smoked cigarettes for 20 years, the effects don't cease the day you stop. Similarly, the effects of a good, low-fat diet are cumulative over many years. Aha, you say, I'm 40 now and I've been eating greasy hamburgers since I was six, so what do I do now? Obviously it would have been nice to be on a low-fat diet one's whole life as a breast cancer preventative, but we can only do what we can do right now. Suffice it to say that a low-fat diet is important as emphasized in the chapter on Nutrition, especially by lowering estrogen levels.

The less exposure your breasts have to estrogen over a shorter period of time, the lower your chances of developing breast cancer.

We know that women who start ovulating (having menstrual periods) at an earlier age (such as nine or ten) have a higher risk for breast cancer because, in effect, they have a longer exposure to estrogen in their lives than women who start ovulating much later, i.e., at 14 or even 16. But do we have any control over this? Apparently so. It has been shown that girls who participate in regular exercise at an early age may actually delay the onset of menarche (beginning of menstrual periods), and thereby decrease the lifelong risk by decreasing estrogen exposure to the breasts.

What about pregnancy? It has been generally found that women who have a pregnancy before age 30 have a lower risk for breast cancer, and those getting pregnant in their late thirties may have an increased risk. Why is this? It has been suggested, though not definitely proved, that this may be related to the length of time the breasts have been exposed to the estrogen of the menstrual cycle. The theory seems to indicate that it is the developing breast in the young woman that is most susceptible to external influences such as estrogen, diet, radiation, and alcohol, and that the "precancerous" changes in the fully mature breasts of a 40 year old have already been set in place. Perhaps that is why the estrogen stimulation of a pregnancy may have a deleterious effect on the woman who gets pregnant for the first time late in life. Remember--this has been suggested by research but not proven.

So let's get back to basics. Hormones have been covered in their own chapter; but it must be emphasized that hormones, after genetic risk factors, are probably the next most important risk factor in developing breast cancer. To summarize, the longer your breasts are exposed to estrogen at high levels, the apparent greater risk for breast cancer. So the theory goes that the more menstrual cycles you have in your lifetime, the higher your risk. Late menarche and early menopause--good; early menarche, late menopause--bad If exercise and activity can delay onset of menarche--good! Then what about removal of the ovaries to induce menopause and lower estrogen? Rather a radical treatment since we can now use medications to achieve almost the same effect. Obviously, the positive effects of hormone support in preventing osteoporosis and heart disease must be weighed in this equation, and the complexity of placing a woman on appropriate levels of hormones (estrogen and progesterone-type birth control to prevent ovulation) to regulate her estrogen output is difficult and very individualized. Your own gynecologist or primary physician can discuss this with you in more detail depending on your own overall risk factors.

Well then there's Tamoxifen. In simplified terms, it's a drug that blocks estrogen release in women. An important clinical trial compared the incidence of breast cancer in certain high risk groups of women, half of which were taking tamoxifen and half placebo (no medication as a control). The study had to be stopped after a few years because the incidence of breast cancer in the tamoxifen group was significantly lower than the control group, and the project directors felt it would be unethical to continue and not place all women who wanted or needed it, on Tamoxifen. We have talked about tamoxifen and risk factors, and the "Gail Mode" risk assessment elsewhere.

Prophylactic mastectomy has a chapter of its own and has been shown in most instances to be too radical and not a major addition to the breast cancer prevention armamentarium. However, some women have a severe cancer phobia (fear), and this operation may have a place for them. But as I have mentioned in a previous chapter, even with a prophylactic mastectomy, some breast tissue always remains, and there is always (although very small) a chance to develop breast cancer.

The most recent experimental work has been in the area of gene therapy. We have discussed the genetics of breast cancer and potential of gene therapy in the Genetics chapter, and new inroads are being made now in this very interesting field. In the next few years we will not only be able to screen high risk women for oncogenes and genetic abnormalities, but also be able to treat the abnormalities and have an impact on breast cancer development.

Another new area for research is that of angiogenesis. For a tumor to grow beyond a certain size it needs nutrients and these are supplied by the tumor causing new blood vessels (angiogenesis) to grow and suffuse the cancer with blood and "building materials". New drugs are being developed which inhibit or prevent the growth of these new blood vessels, thereby stunting or stopping the further growth of the tumor.

Prevention of breast cancer, as you can see, is a complex area in which the Comprehensive Breast Center will focus more attention as newer and better cancer preventatives are developed, so that we do not have to treat existing disease, but can take a step forward by stepping backward and preventing the disease from occurring in the first place.

Chapter 33
THE ARGUMENTS
FOR AND AGAINST
PROPHYLACTIC MASTECTOMY

I n the past year, several articles have appeared in prestigious medical journals and at lectures given in conferences about the value and significance of removing both breasts in women who have a high risk to develop breast cancer. The basic premise of these articles is that women who have their breasts removed will have a lower risk for the development of breast cancer. You might say, "That sounds ridiculous!". If you remove the breasts, then the incidence of breast cancer should be zero. Unfortunately, regardless of how complete a surgeon feels his mastectomy has been, a small amount of breast tissue always remains, and even this small amount of tissue has the potential for developing cancer. In recognizing this, the discussants emphasize that in the selected patients studied, the reduction in the incidence of breast cancer is at least 90%--a very significant number. Well, that's easy enough. If you have a relatively high risk for breast cancer, why not have both breasts removed? Unfortunately, there are many factors which come into play, not least among them being the fact that most physicians and patients do not have an accurate assessment of the risk for breast cancer, and do not have a realistic view as to what this means for their patients or themselves.

So in this chapter, I want to briefly discuss some of the issues surrounding this rather extreme and radical approach to breast cancer prevention. We have discussed the Gail Model risk assessment studies elsewhere, and basically this takes into consideration the onset of menses (when you start having periods), the age when you have you first child, the number of biopsies you have had, and the number, if any, of breast cancers in your immediate family. A risk number is arrived at, and this places a woman into a high, intermediate, or low risk group for developing cancer of the breast. Also, recent studies have found that some women have the BRCA1 and BRCA2 genes which place them at a much higher risk for the development of cancer. The women who fall into the highest risk group are the ones who have been counseled about the possible bilateral prophylactic mastectomies. At the outset, I want to emphasize that there are no conclusive studies to date which support this very radical approach, but there may be instances when a woman, after extensive discussion and counseling, may opt for this procedure.

Remember we are living in an era when the diagnostic capabilities offered by mammography are excellent, and together with breast self-exam and ultrasound, most lesions of the breast can be "picked up" at a very early stage when cure is in the very high 90% range. In women who are at high risk for development of breast cancer, there may be a place for mammography every six months along with frequent careful doctor examinations. Even if the risk were 50% or higher, we should note that of every 100 women undergoing prophylactic mastectomies, half of them would never develop cancer and would be having the procedure and its concomitant physical, social and psychological aftereffects. And we must note that many physicians do not have the expertise and experience to correctly assess a woman's true risk. Having three family members develop breast cancer in their seventies is very much different than if they develop the cancer when in their late twenties or thirties. Many of the reviews indicated that the studies were flawed because of the wide diversity of information and opinion as to what represented true high risk individuals, and many women were unduly "frightened" into having procedures performed which were unwarranted. So what are these "high risk" category criteria? The complete assessment will need to be done by a trained oncologist, but I will give some of the criteria here.

1. Presence of BRCA 1 and BRCA 2 genes.
2. One or more relatives with breast cancer.
3. Relatives who have had breast cancer at an early age.
4. Family history of ovarian cancer.
5. Bilateral breast cancer.
6. Rare breast cancer in male family members.

Others who would fall into the category of possible candidates for bilateral prophylactic mastectomy are:

1. Severe Cancerophobic individuals.
2. High risk women whose mammograms are so dense that screening mammograms cannot be adequately evaluated.
3. Women who have already had one or more lumpectomies, and "don't want to deal with this anymore".

I must, however, stress that this topic of prophylactic mastectomy brings forth many divergent opinions, and the literature is replete with an absence of factual data and uncontrolled and retrospective studies. (This means that the results were often studies obtained "after the fact" rather than designing a prospective or "planned in advance" study). Prophylactic mastectomy may indeed lower the incidence of breast cancer but at present, there is very little hard evidence and data to support recommending this to all but a very few women. And before going ahead with any surgery this radical, I strongly recommend that you have yourself evaluated at a Comprehensive Center where your case can be presented to a board of specialists who can weigh and evaluate your particular problems and needs. Recent advances in the use of chemotherapeutic (drug) agents such as tamoxifen as a cancer preventative agent will probably completely replace prophylactic mastectomy in the near future.

Chapter 34
CONCLUSION

Well finally I've brought this whole book to conclusion,
And haven't left too many filled with confusion.
I hope you have found some wisdom and pleasure,
In exploring the subject from measure to measure.

But conclusions can make you feel happy or sad,
Depending on whether they're cheerful or bad.
It has been my intention in content and scope,
That my book would instill you with knowledge and hope.

But the true answer is that I've learned more than you
In creating this volume I've found something new
For I have been able to write on the Breast
In a manner I have always felt would be best.

There is joy in our lives and love in our hearts,
That comes not from facts or figures or charts,
But from doing a thing which can benefit others,
Like the raising of children by fathers and mothers.

So, trite as it seems, 'twas my labor of love,
Which I've given to you, like shedding a glove,
For I, as a surgeon keep my heart in my hands,
As I meet with each patient and heed her demands.

And to those of you who have faced cancer, I've tried
To give you some dignity, passion and pride
For you know that your life will not be the same
Whether faced with successes or failures or fame.

For you have been forced to look with reality,
Just for a moment on your own mortality.
And the trials you have gone through, like forging a knife,
Will make you much stronger the rest of your life.

Many people live their entire lives without ever having their eyes opened. Oh I don't mean they're physically blind, but that they never have a sense of themselves as a member of society. They never really see the world around them or the people around them. Sometimes it takes a catastrophic event in our lives to give us that new vision, that opens our eyes to life and love and people around us. I sincerely hope that you never have a catastrophic event that cannot be overcome, but I wish you all some event which will give you an emotional or spiritual or philosophical awakening while you are still young enough to appreciate it. Why do I mention this in the conclusion of a book about comprehensive breast care and surviving breast cancer? Because it is the passion that will carry you through the low points in your life, and let you see a different side of living. True, most of you will not get breast cancer; but knowing that one out of eight women will get that disease should give you the chance to help others and thereby help yourselves. Those touched by Cancer are in some ways the lucky ones because they can see a new horizon in their lives. Those who will never have cancer can only reach this understanding by becoming involved with those who have. I would hope that the knowledge and resources in this book will impact your life in a positive way, much as working with patients with breast and other diseases has impacted mine.

DRUGS IS DRUGS

There's Nostrums and Curealls, Panaceas and Opiates
There's Physics and Cures, Soporifics, Barbiturates.
But to be a drug dealer I need a good shingle,
So my drugs'll sound good when I tote 'em and mingle.

You see I go 'Ludes, Weed, Grass, Acid and Buttons
Opium, Hash, Dexies, Speed, Dust, and Mushrooms,
Why, there's Uppers and Downers, Junk, Scag, Smack, and Horse
And there's Barbs, Bennies, Thai Sticks, Black Beauties,
                                        and of course,

The ole Crank, Belladona, Nightshade, Purple Haze,
Marijuana, Psychedelics – ah those were the days.
Yes, there's Grass and Charlie and yep, STP
And to finish it off, Reds and ole LSD.

But you see, my big problem is them cancer drugs,
Ain't got no swell names to throw under the rugs.
No dealer I know who sells and collects
Will sell on the street without names he respects.

So I hereby, respectfully, ask cancer drug makers
To come up with names that will bring in some takers.
For example, instead of the drug 5FU
Why don't we rename it Hot Baby Glue.

And wouldn't you want to use Big Mama Sex
Instead of a silly drug Arimidex?
Cisplatin could do better called Whizz Cisser
And Taxol would flourish if we called it Tax Kisser.
So my plea, you dull drug makers (take my advice),
You should start better marketing with drugs that sound nice
And maybe instead of just making your millions,
You'll be just like me, and start raking in billions!

Drugs Used In The Treatment of Breast Cancer
Hormonal Therapy

Drug	Route of Administration	Side effects	
	IV or Oral	Frequent	Rare
Amino-glutethimide	Oral	Rash, lethargy, fatigue, nausea	Headaches, liver toxicity
Arimidex (Anastrozole)	Oral	Hot flashes	
Diethylstilbestrol (DES)	Oral	Weight gain, nausea, increased blood pressure	Blood clots
Halotestin Leuprolide-Lupron	Oral	Skin changes, fluid retention, altered period, lower voice	Nausea and vomiting, liver toxicity
Prednisone	Oral	Fluid retention, mood changes increased appetite, increased blood sugar	Acne, weakness, high blood pressure
Progestins (Megace)	Oral	Weight gain, breast pain, edema	Hair loss, blood clots
Tamoxifen (Novaldex)	Oral	Hot flashes, nausea, menstrual bleeding clear vaginal discharge	Headache, depression, endometrial cancer, blood clots

Chemotherapeutic Agents

Drug	Route of Administration	Side Effects	
	IV or Oral	Frequent	Rare
Carboplatin (Paraplatin)	IV	Low blood count, nausea, vomiting, hair loss	
Chlorambucil (Leukeran)	Oral	Lethargy, low blood count	Hair loss nausea, vomiting
Cisplatin (Platinol, CDDP)	IV	Neuropathy, nephropathy, nausea, vomiting, hair loss	
Cyclophosphamide (Cytoxan)	Oral and IV	Nausea, vomiting, hair loss, low blood count, loss of appetite	Liver problems, hemorrhagic cystitis, (urinary bleeding)
Doxorubicin (Adriamycin)	IV	Hair loss, nausea, vomiting, low blood count, mouth sores, severe skin reaction if infiltrated	Heart, liver problems
Etoposide (VP-16)	IV	Nausea, vomiting, low blood count, hair loss	
Five (5) and fluorouracil (5-FU)	IV	Nausea, vomiting, diarrhea, hair loss, mouth sores, low blood count, loss of appetite	Skin and nail changes, conjunctivitis
Gemzar (gemcitabine)	IV	Nausea, abdominal upset, low blood count	Hair loss
Melphalan (L-PAM)	Oral	Nausea, vomiting, low blood count	Loss of appetite, mouth sores, rash

Methotrexate	IV	Nausea, vomiting, low blood count, mouth sores, ulcers, rashes	Hair loss, liver, lung problems, headache
Mitomycin C	IV	Nausea, vomiting, low blood count	Mouth sores, loss of hair and appetite, kidney damage
Mitoxantrone (Novantrone)	IV	Nausea, vomiting, low blood count, green urine	Hair loss
Taxanes (Taxol, Taxotere)	IV	Nausea, vomiting, low blood count, fluid retention	Numb hands and feet, rash
Thiotepa	IV	Nausea, vomiting, low blood count	Abdominal pain loss of appetite, hair loss, headache
Vinblastine (Velban)	IV	Nausea, vomiting, hair loss, low blood count	Numbness, weakness, tingling hands and feet
Vincristine	IV	Hair loss, headache, constipation, numbness and tingling of hands and feet, IV site pain, severe skin reaction if infiltrated	Depression, insomnia, muscle and jaw pain
Vinorelbine Tartrate (Navelbine)	IV	Low blood count, neuropathy	Nausea, hair loss

Common Drug Combinations for Breast Cancer

CAF   cytoxan, adriamycin, 5 fluorouracil
CFP   cytoxan, 5 fluorouracil, prednisone
CMF   cytoxan, methotrexate, 5 fluorouracil
CMFVP cytoxan, methotrexate, 5 fluorouracil, vincristine, prednisone
FAC   5 fluorouracil, adriamycin, cytoxan
TAC   Taxane, adriamycin, cytoxan

Antibodies to Cancer

Herceptin	Antibody to cancer cells that over express HER-2/neu	Complications include cardiac (congestive heart failure), nausea, rash, headaches

Medications Used in the Management of Treatment Complications

Nausea	Osteoporosis	Low Red Blood Cell Count	Low White Blood Cell Count	Low Platelet Count
Compazine	Aredia	Epogen	Neupogen	Thrombopoietin
Decadron	Phosphamax	Procrit	Leukine	Neumega
Kytril	Evista			
Reglan	(Raloxifene)			
Zofran				
Anzemet				

RESOURCES
REGIONAL SUPPORT ORGANIZATIONS FOR CANCER AND BREAST CANCER PATIENTS

This resource list is by no means comprehensive. It contains the major resources for you to get information about breast care and breast cancer management. In addition, you can use the facilities of your local American Cancer Society information center and the Internet:

American Cancer Society (ACS)*.
Many free booklets about cancer and normal breast information. ACS National Office, 1599 Clifton Rd. NE, Atlanta, GA 30829--4251. (800) ACS-2345.
American College of Radiology.
Provides Mammography information and lists accredited facilities. (800) 227-5463.
American College of Surgeons.
Names of Board Certified Surgeons in your area. 55 East Erie St., Chicago, IL 60611. (312) 664-4050.
American Society of Clinical Oncology (ASCO).
Information to find specialists in cancer.
American Society of Plastic and Reconstructive Surgeons (ASPRS).
Information about plastic and reconstructive surgery, and lists of Board Certified Plastic Surgeons in your area. 444 East Algonquin Rd., Arlington Heights, IL 60005. (800) 635-0635.
International Cancer Alliance (ICA).
Offers "Cancer Therapy Review" information about cancer and clinical trials. (800) 422-7361.
Komen Alliance and Susan G. Komen Foundation.
Information on research, education, diagnosis, and treatment of breast disease. Susan G. Komen Foundation, Occidental Tower, 5005 LBJ Freeway, Suite 370, Dallas, TX 75224. (214) 450-1777.

Look Good--Feel Better.
Sponsored by ACS and National Cosmetology Association. Helps women deal with changes in their appearance secondary to cancer treatment. See ACS (800) 395-LOOK.
National Alliance of Breast Cancer Organizations (NABCO).
Information and news articles. NABCO, 9 East 37th St. 10th floor, New York, NY 10016. (212) 719-0154.
National Cancer Institute (NCI), Cancer Information Service (CIS).
General cancer information. Office of Cancer Communications, NCI, Building 31, Room 10 A 18, Bethesda, MD 20205. (800) 4-CANCER.
National Council Against Health Fraud
Just what it says! or Dr. John Renner, Consumer Health Information Research Institute, 3521 Broadway, Kansas City, MO 64111. (800) 821-6671.
National Lymphedema Network (NLN).
Broad scope of information about lymphedema and treatment centers. NLN, 2211 Post Street, Suite 404, San Francisco, CA 94115-3427. (415) 921-1306. (800) 541-3259.
National Surgical Adjuvant Breast and Bowel Project (NSABP).
Information of clinical trials and physicians in your area. 3550 Terrance Street, Room 914, Pittsburgh, PA 15261 (412) 648-9720.
National Women's Health Information Center (NWHIC).
A division of U.S. Public Health Service, general and breast cancer information. 1325 G Street NW, Washington, DC 20005. (800) 994-WOMAN.
Physician Data Query (PDQ).
Cancer information database of the NCI-access by computer with modem. Call NCI (800) 4-CANCER.
Reach to Recovery.
Sponsored by ACS-women with breast cancer interact with new patients providing guidance and information and support. See American Cancer Society.
Y-Me National Organization for Breast Cancer.
Education, counseling and support group information. (800) 221-2141.

* Reprinted with the kind permission of the American Cancer Society.

CHARTERED DIVISIONS
OF AMERICAN CANCER SOCIETY

A listing of legally recognized chartered Divisions of the American Cancer Society:

- Eastern Division, Inc. – 2600 US Highway I, North Brunswick, NJ 08902-6001
- Florida Division, Inc, - 3709 West Jetton Avenue, Tampa, FL 33629-5146
- Great Lakes Division, Inc. - 1205 East Saginaw Street, Lansing, MI 48906
- Heartland Division, Inc. - 100 Pennsylvania Ave., Kansas City, MO 64105
- Illinois Division, Inc. - 77 East Monroe Street, Chicago, IL 60603-5795
- Mid-Atlantic Division, Inc. - 4240 Park Place Court, Glen Allen, VA 23060
- Mid-South Division, Inc. - 504 Brookwood Blvd., Birmingham, AL 35209-6802
- Midwest Division, Inc. - 3316 West 66th Street, Minneapolis, MN 55435
- New England Division, Inc, - 30 Speen Street, Framingham, MA 01701-9376
- Ohio Division, Inc.-5555 Frantz Road, Dublin, OH 43017
- Pennsylvania Division, Inc. - Route 422 and Sipe Ave., Hershey, PA 17033-0897
- Rocky Mountain Division, Inc. - 2255 South Oneida, Denver, CO 80224
- Southeast Division, Inc. - 2200 Lake Boulevard, Atlanta, GA 30319
- Southwest Division, Inc. - 2929 East Thomas Road, Phoenix, AZ 85016
- Texas Division, Inc. - 2433 Ridgepoint Dr., Austin, TX 78754
- Northwest Division, Inc. - 2120 First Ave. North, Seattle. WA 98109-1140

- California Division, Inc. –1710 Webster Street, Oakland, CA 94612

COMPREHENSIVE CANCER CENTERS

Below is a list of the NCI-designated cancer centers. Additional information about the Cancer Centers Program can be found on the Cancer Centers Branch Web site at http://www.nci.nih.gov/cancercenters/ on the Internet.

Information about referral procedures, treatment costs, and services available to patients can be obtained from the individual cancer centers listed below.

ALABAMA
University of Alabama at Birmingham
Comprehensive Cancer Center*
Lurleen B. Wallace Tumor Institute
Room 237
1824 Sixth Avenue South
Birmingham, AL 35294-3300
(800) UAB-0933 (800-822-0933)
(205) 975-8222
http://www.ccc.uab.edu/

ARIZONA
University of Arizona Cancer Center*
1515 North Campbell Avenue
Post Office Box 245024
Tucson, AZ 85724
(800) 622-COPE (800-622-2673)
(520) 626-6044
http://www.azcc.arizona.edu

CALIFORNIA
USC/Norris Comprehensive
Cancer Center and Hospital
1441 Eastlake Avenue

Los Angeles, CA 90033-0800
(800) USC-CARE (800-872-2273)
(323) 865-3000
http://ccnt.hsc.usc.edu
cainfo@uscnorris.com (For general information)
UCLA's Jonsson Comprehensive Cancer Center
University of California at Los Angeles
Box 951781
684 Factor Building
Los Angeles, CA 90095-1781
(800) 825-2631
(310) 825-5268
http://www.cancer.mednet.ucla.edu
info@jccc.medsch.ucla.edu
City of Hope National Medical Center
Beckman Research Institute
1500 East Duarte Road
Duarte, CA 91010-3000
(800) 826-HOPE (800-826-4673, New Patient Services office)
(800) 678-9990 (CancerConnection ® service for general cancer
  questions)
(626) 359-8111
http://www.cityofhope.org/
cancerconnection@coh.org (For cancer-related questions)
Chao Family Comprehensive Cancer Center*
University of California at Irvine
Building 23, Route 81
101 The City Drive
Orange, CA 92868
(714) 456-8200
http://www.ucihs.uci.edu/cancer/
University of California, San Diego Cancer Center
9500 Gilman Drive, Mail Code 0658
La Jolla, CA 92093-0658
(619) 822-1222
(619) 822-0207
http://cancer.ucsd.edu

COLORADO
University of Colorado Cancer Center
Box E 190 4200 East Ninth Avenue
Denver, CO 80262
(303) 372-1550
http://www.uchsc.edu/chancllr/UCCC/UCCC.html

CONNECTICUT
Yale Cancer Center
Yale University School of Medicine
333 Cedar Street
New Haven, CT 06520-8028
(203) 785-4095 (Administrative Offices)
http://www.info.med.yale.edu/ycc/

DISTRICT OF COLUMBIA
Lombardi Cancer Center
Georgetown University Medical Center
3800 Reservoir Road, NW
Washington, DC 20007
(202) 784-4000
http://lombardi.georgetown.edu/

FLORIDA
**H. Lee Moffitt Cancer Center & Research Institute
at the University of South Florida**
12902 Magnolia Drive
Tampa, FL 33612-9497
(813) 972-HOPE (813-972-4673)
http://www.moffitt.usf.edu/

HAWAII
Cancer Research Center of Hawai'i
University of Hawai'i
1236 Lauhala Street
Honolulu, HI 96813
(808) 586-3010
http://www2.hawaii.edu/crch/

ILLINOIS
The Robert H. Lurie Cancer Center
Northwestern University
Olson Pavilion 8250
710 North Fairbanks Court
Chicago, IL 60611-3013
(312) 908-5250
http://www.nums.nwu.edu/lurie/index.html
University of Chicago Cancer Research Center
5841 South Maryland Avenue
Chicago, IL 60637-1470
(888) 824-0200 (For new patients)
(773) 702-9200
http://www-uccrc.bsd.uchicago.edu/

MARYLAND
The John Hopkins Oncology Center
600 North Wolfe Street
Baltimore, MD 21287-8943
(410) 955-8964 (For new patients)
http://ww2.ined.jhu.edu/cancerctr/

MASSACHUSETTS
Dana-Farber Cancer Institute*
44 Binney Street
Boston, MA 02115
(800) 320-0022 (For adult patients)
(888) PediOnc (888-733-4662, For patients under 18 years of age)
(617) 632-3000 (Ask for patient information)
http://www.dfci.harvard.edu/site1/otherindex.asp

MICHIGAN
Barbara Ann Karmanos Cancer Institute*
Wertz Clinical Cancer Center
4100 John R
Detroit, MI 48201-1379
(800) KARMANOS (800-527-6266)
(888) KARMANOS (888-527-6266 Physicians' line)

http://www.karmanos.org/
info@karmanos. org
**University of Michigan
Comprehensive Cancer Center**
1500 East Medical Center Drive
Ann Arbor, MI 48109-0843
(800) 865-1125
http://www.cancer.med.umich.edu/
www.cancer@umich.edu

MINNESOTA
Mayo Clinical Cancer Center
200 First Street, SW.
Rochester, MN 55905
(507) 284-9589
http://www.mayo.edu/cancercenter/
University of Minnesota Cancer Center
Box 806
420 Delaware Street, SE.
Minneapolis, MN 55455
(612) 624-8484
http://www.cancer.umn.edu/

NEW HAMPSHIRE
Norris Cotton Cancer Center*
Dartmouth-Hitchcock Medical Center
One Medical Center Drive
Lebanon, NH 03756-0001
(800) 639-6918
(603) 650-5527
http://nccc.hitchcock.org/
Norris.Cotton.Cancer.Center@Dartmouth.edu

NEW JERSEY
The Cancer Institute of New Jersey
Robert Wood Johnson Medical School
195 Little Albany Street
New Brunswick, NJ 08901

(732) 235-6777
http://130.219.231.104/

NEW YORK
Memorial Sloan-Kettering Cancer Center
1275 York Avenue
New York, NY 10021
(800) 525-2225
http://www.mskcc.org
Roswell Park Cancer Institute
Elm and Carlton Streets
Buffalo, NY 14263-0001
(800) ROSWELL (800-767-9355)
http://rpci.med.buffalo.edu/external.html
Kaplan Comprehensive Cancer Center
New York University Medical Center
550 First Avenue
New York, NY 10016
(212) 263-6485
http://kccc-www.med.nyu.edu
Herbert Irving Comprehensive Cancer Center
Columbia University
Room 435, Sixth Floor
Milstein Hospital Building
177 Fort Washington Avenue
New York, NY 10032
(212) 305-8610
http://www.ccc.columbia.edu/
Albert Einstein Comprehensive Cancer Center
Albert Einstein College of Medicine
1300 Morris Park Avenue
Bronx, NY 10461
(718) 430-2302
http:/www.ca.aecom.yu.edu/
aeccc@aecom.yu.edu
University of Rochester Cancer Center**
Box 704
601 Elmwood Avenue

Rochester, NY 14642
(716) 275-4911
http://www.urmc.rochester.edu/strong/
cancer/cancerpg.htm

NORTH CAROLINA
Duke Comprehensive Cancer Center
Duke University Medical Center
Box 3843
Durham, NC 27710
(919) 684-3377
http://www.Canctr.mc.duke.edu/
UNC Lineberger Comprehensive Cancer Center
University of North Carolina Chapel Hill
School of Medicine
Campus Box 7295
102 West Drive
Chapel Hill, NC 27599-7295
(919) 966-3036
(919) 966-1101
http://cancer.med.unc.edu/

NORTH CAROLINA
Comprehensive Cancer Center at Wake Forest University
Battist Medical Center
Medical Center Boulevard
Winston-Salem, NC 27157-1082
(336) 716-2075
http://www.bgsm.edu/cancer/

OHIO
The Ohio State University Comprehensive Cancer Center
The Arthur G. James Cancer Hospital and Research Institute
300 West 10th Avenue
Columbus, OH 43210-1240
(800) 293-5066 (The James Line)
http://www-cancer.med.Ohio-state.edu/

Ireland Cancer Center
University Hospitals of Cleveland
11100 Euclid Avenue
Cleveland, OH 44106-5065
(800) 641-2422
(216) 844-5432
http://www.uhhs.com/uhc/cancer/index.html

OREGON
Oregon Health Sciences University
3181 Southwest Sam Jackson Park Road
Portland, OR 97201-3098
(503) 494-9000
http://www.ohsu.edu/

PENNSYLVANIA
Fox Chase Cancer Center
7701 Burholme Avenue
Philadelphia, PA 19111
(888) FOXCHASE (888-369-2427, Patient services line)
(215) 728-6900
http://www.fccc.edu/
University of Pennsylvania Cancer Center
15th Floor, Penn Tower Hotel
3400 Spruce Street
Philadelphia, PA 19104-4383
(800) 383-UPCC (800-383-8722)
(215) 662-6364
http://cancer.med.upenn.edu/
University of Pittsburgh Cancer Institute
Information & Referral Service
Suite 206
Iroquois Building
3600 Forbes Avenue
Pittsburgh, PA 15213-3410
(800) 237-4PCI (800-237-4724)
http://www.upci.upmc.edu/
Kimmel Cancer Center

Thomas Jefferson University
Suite 1014
College Building
1025 Walnut Street
Philadelphia, PA 19107
(800) JEFF-NOW (800-533-3669. Jefferson Cancer Network)
(800) 654-5984 (Jefferson Cancer Network toll-free number forhearing and speech impaired callers)
(800) 4-CNETWORK (800-426-3895, for physician referrals)
http://www.kcc.tju.edu/

TENNESSEE
St. Jude Children's Research Hospital
332 North Lauderdale Street
Memphis, TN 38105-0318
(888) 226-4343 (Physician referral line)
(901) 495-3300
http://www.stjude.org/
info@stjude.org (For general information)
Vanderbilt Cancer Center
Vanderbilt University
649 Medical Research Building II
Nashville, TN 37232-6838
(800) 811-8480
(615) 936-1782
http://www.mc.Vanderbilt.Edu/vumc/centers/cancer/

TEXAS
The University of Texas M.D. Anderson Cancer Center
1515 Holcombe Boulevard
Houston, TX 77030
(800) 392-1611
http://www.mdanderson.org/
San Antonio Cancer Institute
8122 Datapoint Drive
San Antonio, TX 78229-3264
(210) 616-5590
http://www.ccc.saci.org/

UTAH
Huntsman Cancer Institute
University of Utah
Room 2100
15 North 2030 East
Salt Lake City, UT 84112-5330
(800) 488-2422
(801)581-6365
http://www.hci.utah.edu/

VERMONT
Vermont Cancer Center
University of Vermont
Medical Alumni Building
Burlington, VT 05405-0068
(802) 656-4414
http://www.vtmednet.org/vcc
vcc@uvm.edu

VIRGINIA
Massey Cancer Center
Virginia Commonwealth University
401 College Street
Post Office Box 980037
Richmond, VA 23298-0037
(804) 828-0450
http://views.vcu.edu/mcc/
The Cancer Center at University of Virginia
Post Office Box 334
Charlottesville.VA 22908
(800) 223-9173
(804) 924-9333
http://www.med.virginia.edu/medcntr/cancer/home.html

WASHINGTON
Fred Hutchinson Cancer Research Center
FM-252
1100 Fairview Avenue North

Post Office Box 19024
Seattle, WA 98109-1024
(800) 804-8824
206) 667-4324
http://www.fhcrc.org/
hutchdoc@fhcrc.org (Patient information)

WISCONSIN
University of Wisconsin Comprehensive Cancer Center
600 Highland Avenue
Madison, WI 53792-0001
(800) 622-8922
(608) 263-8600
http://www.medsch.wisc.edu/cancer/homepage.html

* Reprinted with the kind permission of the National Cancer Institute.

***

CANCER CENTERS
SUPPORTED BY THE NATIONAL CANCER INSTITUTE

The Burnham Institute
La Jolla, California

Armand Hammer Center for Cancer Biology, Salk Institute
La Jolla, California

Purdue Cancer Center, Purdue University
West Lafayette, Indiana

The Jackson Laboratory
Bar Harbor, Maine

Center for Cancer Research, Massachusetts Institute of Technology
Cambridge, Massachusetts

Eppley Institute, University of Nebraska Medical Center

Omaha, Nebraska

Cold Spring Harbor Laboratory
Cold Spring Harbor, New York

American Health Foundation
New York, New York

Wistar Institute
Philadelphia, Pennsylvania

McArdle Laboratory for Cancer Research, University of Wisconsin
Madison, Wisconsin

***

SOURCES OF
NATIONAL CANCER INSTITUTE INFORMATION

Cancer Information Service
Toll-free: 1-800-4-CANCER (1-800-422-6237)
TTY: 1-800-332-8615

NCI Online

Internet
Use http://www.nci.nih.gov to reach NCI's Web site.

CancerMail Service
To obtain a contents list, send e-mail to cancermail@icicc.nci.nih.gov
with the word "help" in the body of the message.

CancerFax® fax on demand service
Dial 301-402-5874 and listen to recorded instructions.

GLOSSARY

Now why would anyone want to write a poem about a glossary?
You'd think, as others will, that this is just a bit propossary.
For after all its just a bunch of high fallutin words,
A lot of which you probably think are really quite absurd.

But in this glossary are hidden the secrets of the ages
The magic of eternal youth you'll find on certain pages.
But I have mixed these secrets up (with poems absurd and funny),
Which I will only tell to you for lots and lots of money.

Now you may say, I'm quite a cad, to do it just for dollars
But let's be honest, who is going to iron all my collars?
I'm just a pragmatist at heart, if I may be so bold,
This is the glossary Olympics and I'm going for the Gold.

So flutter through this list of words, pretend you know them all
Look up the definitions and remember to stand tall;
So when your friends are congregating, sipping tea with scones,
Blurt out everything you know (you'll shock 'em to their bones).

And when they ask you where you got your mastery of language
Just smile and raise your eyebrows; and take a bite out of you
sandwage.

GLOSSARY

Abscess: A pocket of pus that forms when the body attempts to wall off an infection.

Acute: Of short duration (as opposed to chronic), severe, sharp (as pain).

Adenocarcinoma: Cancer whose origin is the gland forming tissue – i.e., breast cancer.

Adjuvant Chemotherapy: Anticancer drugs used to treat a tumor before it has spread to prevent or delay recurrence and used in conjunction with surgery and/or radiation.

Adriamycin: *See* Doxorubicin

Alopecia: Loss of hair seen with some types of chemotherapy.

Aminoglutethimide: A hormonal drug therapy for breast cancer.

Androgen: Hormone responsible for male characteristics.

Aneuploid: A measure of the abnormal amount of DNA in a cell often correlating with more severe cancer.

Anzemet: An anti-nausea medication

Aredia: A drug for treating, preventing osteoporosis.

Areola: The pigmented tissue surrounding the nipple.

Arimidex: A hormonal drug therapy for breast cancer.

Aromatase Inhibitors: Hormones that kill cancer cells by blocking estrogen.

Aspiration: The removal of fluid from a cyst; the removal of cells from a lump using a needle and syringe.

Atypia: Abnormality in a cell.

Atypical Hyperplasia: Not cancer, but abnormal changes in a cell.

Augmentation: Increase in size as with augmentation mammoplasty.

Autologous: From the same person.

Axilla: The armpit.

Axillary Lymph Nodes: Lymph nodes found in the armpit.

Benign: Not cancerous.

Biopsy: The removal of tissue for examination.

Blue Nodes: *See* Sentinel Node Biopsy - the nodes found using the blue dye technique.

Bone Marrow: The soft fatty tissue that fill the cavity of most bones and produces blood cells.

Bone Scan: A radiological test to determine if there is evidence of cancer in the bones.

Bone Marrow Transplantation: UA technique used after very high dose chemotherapy to replenish the bone marrow.

BRCA1 and BRCA2 genes: Genes that when altered, indicate an inherited high susceptibility to developing breast cancer.

Calcifications: Small inclusions of calcium in tissue which can be seen on mammograms.

Cancer: A general name for many diseases in which abnormal cells grow, invade, and destroy healthy tissue and may spread throughout the body.

Cancer Committee: A group of professionals who meet regularly to discuss cancer cases and decide upon therapy.

Carboplatin (paraplatin): Chemotherapeutic drug for breast cancer.

Carcinoembryonic Antigen (CEA): A blood test sometimes used to evaluate the effectiveness of a cancer treatment.

Carcinogen: Something that can cause cancer.

Carcinoma: Cancer arising from epithelial tissue (skin, glands, parts of organs), i.e., breast cancer.

Carcinoma in situ: Cancer that is confined the area where it developed and has not yet spread to adjacent tissue.

Cellulitis: Infection of the soft tissues (i.e., skin).

Chemotherapy: The treatment of disease with drugs; descriptive of the treatment of cancer with cytotoxic drugs.

Chlorambucil (Leukeran): Chemotherapeutic drug for breast cancer.

Chromosomes: String-like structure found in the nucleus of a cell and containing genes.

Chronic: Lasting a long time (as opposed to Acute).

Cisplatin (Platinol): Chemotherapeutic drug for breast cancer.

Clear Margins: Describing the normal, cancer-free tissue margin of a surgical specimen.

Clinical Stage: A determination of the activity of a tumor by pathology, measurement, and symptoms.

Colostrum: The liquid discharge from the nipple just prior to milk production.

Comedo: A more aggressive type of DCIS.

Compazine: An anti-nausea medication.

Contracture: A scar tissue that may develop especially around a breast implant causing firmness.

Core Needle Biopsy: Taking tissue from the breast using a large needle instead of surgery.

Cribriform: Type of DCIS with a punched-out appearance.

Cyclophosphamide (Cytoxan): Chemotherapeutic drug for breast cancer.

Cysts: Fluid-filled sacs.

Cystosarcoma Phylloides: An unusual type of breast disease which may be malignant.

Cytology: Study of cells under a microscope.

Cytoxan: *See* Cyclophosphamide.

Danocrine; Danazol: A drug used to block hormones used in endometriosis and in severe cases of cystic breast disease.

Decadron: Steroid used for treatments of nausea and inflammatory disease.

Decongestive Therapy: A treatment modality for lymphedema.

Diagnostic Mammogram: X-ray of the breast in a woman who has symptoms such as a lump or whose screening mammogram has an abnormality.

Diethylstilbestrol (DES): A hormonal drug therapy for breast cancer.

Diploid: Normal amount of cellular DNA, two sets of chromosomes, associated with better prognosis in breast cancer.

Doxorubicin (adriamycin): Chemotherapeutic drug for breast cancer.

Ducts and Ductal Cells: Tubes or channels in the breast; their cells.

Ductal Carcinoma in situ (DCIS): *See* Carcinoma in situ.

Edema: Swelling due to an abnormal accumulation of fluid in tissue or cells.

Embolus or Embolism: Blood clot which can travel to the lungs; a plug of tumor cells in a vessel.

Epogen: Drug to treat low red blood cell count.

Estrogen: Female sex hormones - produced in ovaries, placenta, adrenal glands, fat or artificially produced; responsible for secondary sex characteristics in women.

Estrogen Receptor: An area in a cell where estrogen may attach. If a cancer is Estrogen receptor positive, it is sensitive to this hormone.

Etoposide (VP-16): Chemotherapeutic drug for breast cancer.

Evista: *See* Raloxifene.

Excisional Biopsy: Complete removal of a mass or tumor.

Expander: An implant, usually saline, which is placed under the skin and gradually enlarged to prepare for placement of a permanent breast implant.

False Negative: A mammogram or other diagnostic procedure which appears normal and misses a cancer when it is present.

False Positive: A mammogram or diagnostic procedure which appears to show cancer when there is none.

Fat Necrosis: Lumpy fatty breast material usually secondary to trauma or surgery.

Fibroadenoma: A benign breast tumor usually with a rubbery feeling; usually in young women.

Fibrocystic Disease: A vague, generalized term for non-cancerous lumpiness and irregularities of the breast.

Fine Needle Aspiration: Obtaining fluid or tissue using a very slender needle.

Five Fluorouracil (5-FU): Chemotherapeutic drug for breast cancer.

Frozen Section: A fast diagnostic test of tissue by the pathologist for determining if a mass has cancer. The tissue is frozen and sliced so it can be examined under a microscope.

Gail Model: A way of determining risk for breast cancer.

Galactocele: Milk cyst - usually occurring in a nursing mother.

Gemzar (gemcitabine): Chemotherapeutic drug for breast cancer.

Gene: A segment of a DNA molecule on a chromosome responsible for inherited diseases.

Genetic Change: A change in the gene which may lead to disease.

Gynecomastia: Abnormal enlargement of the male breast.

Halotestin: A hormonal drug therapy for breast cancer.

Haploid: Having only half the number of chromosomes as the normal cell.

Hematoma: A collection of blood or blood clots in a body cavity (such as the breast after biopsy).

HER-2/neu: An oncogene associated with cancer when abnormally expressed.

Histologic Grade: A grading of the cancer by its appearance under the microscope by a pathologist.

Holistic Medicine: An approach to medicine stressing the mind--body entity.

Hormone Replacement Therapy: Hormone-containing medicine to replace or augment the body's own losses or deficit – i.e., estrogen replacement after menopause.

Hormones: Substances produced by glands in the body which have an effect on other tissues.

Hyperplasia: Excessive growth of cells.

Immune System: The body's defense system against internal or external abnormalities such as infection and cancer.

Incisional Biopsy: The surgical removal of only a portion of tissue or mass.

Infections: Growth in the body of micro-organisms such as bacteria and viruses.

Infiltrating Carcinoma or Cancer: *See* cancer; Cancer that has spread beyond the local area to surrounding tissue, lymph nodes or other parts of the body.

Inflammation: The body's response to infection or injury (such as surgery) characterized by heat, redness, swelling, pain (calor, rubor, tumor, dolor in old Latin!).

In Situ: Usually referring to cancer which has not spread beyond its site of origin.

Intraductal Papilloma: A benign tumor that grows in breast duct occasionally causing nipple discharge.

Invasive Cancer: Same as infiltrating carcinoma.

Kytril: An anti-nausea medication.

Lactation: Producing milk.

Latissimus Muscle Flap: Rotation of a muscle to cover a defect after more extensive breast surgery such as mastectomy.

Leukeran: *See* chlorambucil.

Leukine: Drug to treat low white blood cell count.

Lobes, Lobules: Milk producing breast tissue, usually 15-20 lobes, branching to lobules and ending in a milk bulb.

Lobular Carcinoma in situ: Not cancer - a misnomer - when these abnormal cells occur in a breast lobule, there is an increased risk of finding cancer elsewhere in the breast. It is a marker for breast cancer.

Local Control: Removing the local tumor of the breast.

Local Recurrence: Return of cancer in the breast or chest wall area.

Localization Biopsy: Placement of needle by a radiologist using x-rays or ultrasound so that a surgeon can biopsy or remove the abnormal area when no mass can be felt.

L-PAM: *See* Melphalan.

Lumpectomy: Removing abnormal tissue from the breast with a margin of normal tissue around it.

Lupron: A hormonal drug for breast cancer.

Lymphatic System and Lymph Nodes: The tissues and organs in the body that help fight against foreign invaders -- bacteria, cancer. Cancer can sometimes spread to nodes.

Lymphedema: Swelling caused by lymph due to failure of normal lymph circulation resulting in accumulation of lymph in body tissues such as the arm after axillary dissection.

Malignancy: Cancerous condition.

Mammogram: An x-ray of the breast usually done with compression and several views using a special mammogram machine.

Mastectomy: Surgical removal of the breast. There are many different types of mastectomy.

Mastitis: Inflammation or infection of the breast.

Mastodynia: Painful breast.

Mastopexy: Breast lift using plastic surgery.

Megace: A progestin hormonal drug for breast cancer treatment.

Melphalan (L-PAM): Chemotherapeutic drug for breast-cancer.

Menarche: The first menstrual period.

Menopause: "Change of Life"; The gradual or immediate (due to surgery or treatment) cessation of menstruation.

Metastasis: Spread of cancer to another organ.

Methotrexate: Chemotherapeutic drug for breast cancer.

Microcalcifications: Tiny white spots indicating calcium deposits seen on a mammogram which may indicate benign or cancerous conditions.

Micrometastasis: Cancer in other organs or lymph nodes that a pathologist can only detect with special studies.

Mitomycin C: Chemotherapeutic drug for breast cancer.

Mitosis, Mitotic: The process of cell division that causes the reproduction of cells.

Mitoxantrone (Novantrone): Chemotherapeutic drug for breast cancer.

Mutation: Change, usually used when we speak about changes in genes.

Myocutaneous Flap: Consisting of skin, muscle and underlying tissue used by plastic surgeons in reconstructing the breast after major surgery.

Navelbine: *See* Vinorelbine.

Necrosis: Death of tissue.

Needle Biopsy: Use of a needle and syringe to extract cells or fluid.

Neoadjuvant Chemotherapy: Using chemotherapy for treatment of cancer prior to surgery.

Neumega: Drug to treat low platelet counts.

Neupogen: Drug to treat low white blood cell count.

Nipple Discharge: Any fluid discharge from the nipple, clear, cloudy or bloody, not usually a sign of cancer.

Nodular: Lumpy.

Nolvadex: Same as tamoxifen.

Nonpalpable: Can't be felt.

Novantrone: *See* mitoxantrone.

Oncogene: Genes that can cause cancer when activated in the body.

Oncology: The study of tumors; usually referring to cancer.

Osteoporosis: Mineral loss causing weakening of the bones and increased risk for fractures.

Palpation: Using the fingers for examination.

Papillary Cancer: A type of ductal cancer of the breast.

Pathologist: A physician who diagnose diseases by examining tissue either grossly or under a microscope.

Pectoralis Major and Minor: The large muscle masses lying under the breast.

Permanent Section: Tissue processed and examined by the pathologist under a microscope. This preparation usually takes 24 hours as opposed to the rapid frozen section.

Phlebitis: Inflammation of a vein.

Placebo: An inactive substance given in place of real medicine.

Platinol: *See* cisplatin.

Positron Emission Tomography (PET Scan): Another more modern method of x-ray diagnostics.

Postmenopausal: After having gone through the menopause.

Prednisone: Drug used in hormonal therapy (for breast cancer and other diseases).

Premarin: Estrogen sometimes given to women after menopause.

Procrit: Drug used to treat low red blood cell count.

Progesterone: A hormone produced by the ovary which is active in breast development and changes occurring throughout the menstrual cycle.

Prophylactic Mastectomy: Removal of the breast to prevent breast cancer or lower the risk of developing breast cancer evaluate the relative risk of cure or recurrence of
cancer.

Quadrant: One fourth of the breast.

Quadrantectomy: Removal of one-fourth of the breast; a generous lumpectomy or partial mastectomy.

Rad: A unit of Radiation Dose.

Radiation Therapy: Treatment of a portion with radiation to cure or treat or prevent the spread of a cancer.

Raloxifene: Hormonal agent being tested for prevention and use against breast cancer.

Randomized Clinical Trials: A recognized method of studying the effectiveness of a drug treatment, under carefully controlled conditions.

Receptors: An area or substance in a cell that combines with a drug , hormone, or chemical to alter the cell's function.

Recurrence: A return of a cancer after initial treatment and disappearance.

Reglan: An anti-nausea medication.

Remission: Disappearance of a cancer. (No clinical or diagnostic evidence of the tumor).

S Phase: Another measurement of cell division activity used in prognosis of cancer.

Sclerosing Adenosis: A benign breast disease characterized by an excessive growth of tissue in the breast's lobules.

Screening Mammogram: A mammogram done in an asymptomatic woman to detect abnormalities.

Sentinel Node: The first lymph node draining a particular area of the breast. It may not contain cancer.

Sonogram: An ultrasound picture of the breast, sometimes helpful in identifying cysts and as an adjunct to mammography.

Seroma: A collection of fluid in a body cavity -- as at the site of a biopsy or mastectomy.

Staging: An assessment of the cancer by criteria of size, tumor type, node involvement, and presence or absence of metastasis.

Stem Cell: A cell that has the potential to form new bone marrow and produce blood cells.

Stereotactic Localization: *See* Needle Localization. Also, localization by the radiologist while doing a stereotactic biopsy.

Stereotactic Biopsy: A large bore needle biopsy (i.e., of breast), under radiographic visualization when a mass cannot be felt. This is done by a radiologist or surgeon.

Systemic Treatment: Treatment of the entire body, usually with intravenous or oral drugs or in conjunction with radiation therapy.

Tamoxifen: An older drug with a relatively new found use in preventing breast cancer. It is an estrogen blocker and is also used to treat breast cancer.

Taxanes (Taxol, Taxotere): Chemotherapeutic drug for breast cancer.

Thiotepa: Chemotherapeutic drug for breast cancer.

Thrombopoietin: Drug to treat low platelet count.

Toxicity: A measure of the ill-effects of a medicine.

TRAM Flap: A plastic surgical procedure rotating tissue from the abdomen to fill a defect after extensive breast surgery.

Tru-Cut Biopsy: A type of needle biopsy that can be done by the physician in the office.

Tubular Cancer: A type of slower growing, less virulent breast cancer.

Tumor: Any abnormal growth of tissue. A tumor may be benign (non-cancerous) or malignant (cancerous).

Tumor Markers: Proteins made by tumors which can be identified and used in cancer evaluations.

Ultrasound: A diagnostic tool using sound waves to produce images -- another way of evaluating the breast.

Vinblastine (Velban): Chemotherapeutic drug for breast cancer.

Vincristine: Chemotherapeutic drug for breast cancer.

Vinorelbine (Navelbine): Chemotherapeutic drug for breast cancer.

VP-16: *See* etoposide, chemotherapeutic drug for breast cancer.

Zofran: An anti-nausea medication.

INDEX